Overcoming Insomnia

Susan Elliot-Wright is a freelance writer and journalist specializing in health and parenting. Since training as a journalist while raising her two (now grown-up) children, she has written for a number of magazines and newspapers, and is the author of four health information books for teenagers, as well as *Coping with Type 2 Diabetes* (2006), *Living with Heart Failure* (2006) and *Overcoming Emotional Abuse* (2007), all published by Sheldon Press. She and her husband live in Sheffield, where she is taking a Master's degree in writing. She hopes to divide her energies between producing fiction and non-fiction.

GW00689779

Overcoming Common Problems Series

Selected titles

A full list of titles is available from Sheldon Press,
36 Causton Street, London SW1P 4ST and on our website at
www.sheldonpress.co.uk

The Assertiveness Handbook
Mary Hartley

Assertiveness: Step by Step
Dr Windy Dryden and Daniel Constantinou

Body Language: What You Need to Know
David Cohen

Breaking Free
Carolyn Ainscough and Kay Toon

Calm Down
Paul Hauck

The Candida Diet Book
Karen Brody

Cataract: What You Need to Know
Mark Watts

The Chronic Fatigue Healing Diet
Christine Craggs-Hinton

The Chronic Pain Diet Book
Neville Shone

Cider Vinegar
Margaret Hills

Comfort for Depression
Janet Horwood

The Complete Carer's Guide
Bridget McCall

The Confidence Book
Gordon Lamont

Confidence Works
Gladeana McMahon

Coping Successfully with Pain
Neville Shone

Coping Successfully with Panic Attacks
Shirley Trickett

Coping Successfully with Period Problems
Mary-Claire Mason

Coping Successfully with Prostate Cancer
Dr Tom Smith

Coping Successfully with Ulcerative Colitis
Peter Cartwright

Coping Successfully with Varicose Veins
Christine Craggs-Hinton

Coping Successfully with Your Hiatus Hernia
Dr Tom Smith

Coping Successfully with Your Irritable Bowel
Rosemary Nicol

Coping with Age-related Memory Loss
Dr Tom Smith

Coping with Alopecia
Dr Nigel Hunt and Dr Sue McHale

Coping with Blushing
Dr Robert Edelmann

Coping with Bowel Cancer
Dr Tom Smith

Coping with Brain Injury
Maggie Rich

Coping with Candida
Shirley Trickett

Coping with Chemotherapy
Dr Terry Priestman

Coping with Childhood Allergies
Jill Eckersley

Coping with Childhood Asthma
Jill Eckersley

Coping with Chronic Fatigue
Trudie Chalder

Coping with Coeliac Disease
Karen Brody

Coping with Compulsive Eating
Ruth Searle

Coping with Diabetes in Childhood and Adolescence
Dr Philippa Kaye

Coping with Diverticulitis
Peter Cartwright

Coping with Down's Syndrome
Fiona Marshall

Coping with Dyspraxia
Jill Eckersley

Overcoming Common Problems Series

Overcoming Common Problems Series

Overcoming Common Problems

Overcoming Insomnia

SUSAN ELLIOT-WRIGHT

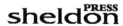

First published in Great Britain in 2008

Sheldon Press
36 Causton Street
London SW1P 4ST

Copyright © Susan Elliot-Wright 2008

All rights reserved. No part of this book may be reproduced or
transmitted in any form or by any means, electronic or mechanical,
including photocopying, recording, or by any information storage and
retrieval system, without permission in writing from the publisher.

The author and publisher have made every effort to ensure that the
external website and email addresses included in this book are correct and
up to date at the time of going to press. The author and publisher are not
responsible for the content, quality or continuing accessibility of the sites.

British Library Cataloguing-in-Publication Data
A catalogue record for this book is available from the British Library

ISBN 978-1-84709-031-7

1 3 5 7 9 10 8 6 4 2

Typeset by Fakenham Photosetting Ltd, Fakenham, Norfolk
Printed in Great Britain by Ashford Colour Press

Produced on paper from sustainable forests

Contents

Note to the reader

This is not a medical book and is not intended to replace advice from your doctor. Consult your pharmacist or doctor if you believe you have any of the symptoms described, and if you think you might need medical help.

Introduction

Around a third of the population has difficulty getting a good night's sleep, and around one in ten people find this has a significant impact on their quality of life. More women than men have trouble sleeping, and it's something that seems to affect more older people. Among the most common sleep difficulties are:

- difficulty getting to sleep;
- frequent waking during the night;
- waking after a couple of hours and having difficulty getting back to sleep;
- early morning waking;
- feeling tired and unrefreshed after sleep.

There may be a single reason why someone can't sleep – pain, for example, or a noisy environment – but there are often a number of contributory factors. These include physical problems such as medical conditions, hormonal changes or side effects of certain medicines; psychological factors such as stress or grief; environmental factors such as an uncomfortable bed or a snoring partner; mental health problems such as depression or anxiety; lifestyle factors such as jet lag; or stimulants such as alcohol, nicotine or caffeine.

Some people suggest that insomnia is a modern issue, and that it is our 24/7 culture that is responsible. We live, after all, in a culture where we can do our banking online at two in the morning, go supermarket shopping at three, and watch a film on television as dawn breaks. Our modern lifestyle means we are also more likely to work at night or do shift work, or to be travelling across time zones, all of which can upset our 'biological clock'.

Before the industrial revolution and the advent of electric light, we were more likely to follow the pattern dictated by our bodies, which would have been to rise at daybreak, work through most of the daylight hours and then to wind down after sunset. There is some debate as to whether our ancestors slept for longer than we do today, but there is evidence to suggest that their sleep patterns were different. It was not uncommon in Northern Europe, for example, to take a nap in the afternoon (a practice still common in some Mediterranean countries), especially in the summer months. During the dark winter months, when people went to bed earlier and woke later, there would often be a period of quiet wakefulness lasting for an hour or more midway through the night. The two periods of sleep were known as 'first sleep' and 'second sleep'.

In the twenty-first century, most people's sleep patterns are dictated by the need to work long hours with few breaks. This means no chance of an afternoon nap during the summer, and as we tend not to go to bed any earlier in the winter and we still have to be up at 7 a.m. to go to work, an hour of wakefulness during the night will make us sleepy and irritable the following day.

There is no doubt that lack of sleep causes problems. Apart from the fact that a badly disturbed night makes us feel awful, it can also be dangerous. You are more likely to make mistakes at work, or to have an accident, if you haven't had enough sleep. Chronic (long-term) insomnia can lead to mental health problems such as depression and can also affect your physical health, weakening your immune system and making you vulnerable to illness and infection. Poor sleep can impact on your relationship, too, making you short-tempered and snappy with your partner for no apparent reason, or because you may feel he or she is partly to blame for your sleeplessness – perhaps your partner snores or moves about a lot during the night.

Given that lack of sleep can make our lives a misery, it is perhaps surprising that relatively few people seek help from their doctor. This may be because they feel that the situation isn't a 'medical' one, that it's not severe enough to warrant a trip to the surgery, or that they should be able to cope with less sleep because a magazine article said they only need seven hours or whatever. Some people may be put off by the idea that all their doctor can do is to prescribe sleeping tablets to which they might become addicted. In fact, there are a number of options for treating sleep difficulties, many of which don't involve any medication at all. Treatment will depend on what is causing your insomnia, but you may be pleasantly surprised to find that there are many steps you can take to improve the quality and quantity of your sleep, with or without seeing your doctor.

The aim of this book is to arm you with the information you need to be able to start addressing your sleep difficulties straight away, so that you begin to feel the benefits as soon as possible. In order to do this, it helps to understand a little about the process of sleep – why we sleep, why we dream and so on. Chapter 1 looks at these questions and also dispels some myths about sleep. Chapter 2 asks 'What is insomnia?' This chapter will help you to recognize your own patterns of sleeping and waking. It explains a little about the body's natural sleep–wake rhythms – what we call 'the body clock' – and shows how these rhythms can easily be upset by our lifestyle.

Chapter 3 looks at why insomnia should not go untreated. The impact on your health, work, social life and relationships can be significant, and your quality of life seriously reduced. The sad thing is, many people don't realize that it is their insomnia that is at the root of some (or many) of their daily problems. This chapter may help you to understand how lack of sleep is affecting your own life.

Chapters 4 and 5 go through the possible causes of insomnia in some detail, suggesting solutions for each, and Chapter 6 looks at general steps you can take to get a better night's sleep. This chapter is packed with advice on things like choosing the right bed, making sure your bedroom is conducive to sleep, what foods or drinks can help you to sleep, what might keep you awake, and so on. This chapter also looks at some of the natural remedies and complementary therapies available so you can make an informed choice when deciding what to try. There are many natural ways to treat insomnia and its causes – so many, in fact, that it can be quite confusing, leaving you wondering which is best. Different approaches work for different people, and it may take some time to find the one that's right for you. There is also a quick reference guide at the end of the chapter with tips for a good night's sleep.

If, despite your best efforts, refreshing sleep still eludes you, it is probably wise to seek medical help. Depending on your history and what is known about your sleep patterns, your doctor may suggest self-help measures, a short course of medication or a referral to a sleep clinic to try and establish what's causing your insomnia. Chapter 7 looks at types of sleeping tablets, the pros and cons of taking them and, if you're already taking them, how to best wean yourself off and still get a good night's sleep. This chapter also explains what a sleep clinic is, and how the experts can help.

Chapter 8 looks briefly at less common sleep disorders such as nightmares, night terrors, sleepwalking, narcolepsy, hypersomnia and sleep paralysis. These are sometimes known as 'parasomnias', which simply means 'dysfunction around sleep'.

The final chapter addresses one of the main causes of lack of sleep in adults – wakeful children! All parents suffer broken nights, especially when their children are babies, but if sleeplessness persists there may be things you can do to improve the situation and help your child – and the rest of the household – to get a decent night's sleep.

Sometimes, especially at four in the morning when your partner, your children and even the dog are all snoozing happily, you may feel you're the only person on the planet who is still awake, watching the clock labour from minute to minute through what seems like an endless night. At these times, it may help you to pick up this book and flick through to the personal stories of others who have had the same experience. Just knowing that you're not the only one can help, but what's really encouraging is to see how many people manage to overcome or at least improve their sleep difficulties and now rarely lie awake half the night in that torturous state of sleepless exhaustion.

I hope this book will help to give you a deeper understanding of sleep and its disorders, and that you will find some ideas on how to tackle your own sleep situation, leading to more restful nights and more relaxed and productive days.

I would like to thank all those who were kind enough to share with me their experiences of sleep and lack of it, and of the investigations and treatments they have undergone in pursuit of refreshing slumber. I bid you all many good nights!

1

Understanding sleep

According to the concise version of the *Oxford English Dictionary*, sleep is 'a regularly recurring condition of body and mind in which the nervous system is inactive, the eyes closed, the postural muscles relaxed, and consciousness practically suspended'. During sleep we stop responding to our surroundings, but this does not mean that everything else stops – sleep is not like simply switching off a light. In fact, quite a lot goes on in our bodies while we're asleep, such as the release of certain hormones, for example, and the laying down of proteins for growth and repair.

Most humans will sleep for at least one period during every 24 hours, and before the early twentieth century this would usually be during the hours of darkness. Our work and sleep patterns back then were also affected by the seasons: we worked more and slept less during the lighter, warmer months than we did in the cold winter months, when we tended to stay indoors after dark, sleeping for longer and generally being less active. This is similar to the pattern adopted by animals that hibernate. With industrialization, however, our work patterns changed in order to meet the demands of industry, and when we started to use electric lighting there was no need for production to halt during the hours of darkness. As a result of this change in work patterns, we were also forced to change our sleep patterns, reordering our lives completely to fit in with the modern world. This means that what we describe as a 'normal' or 'natural' pattern of sleep may not actually be normal or natural at all.

Why do we sleep?

There is still a great deal we don't understand about why we need to sleep, but the main functions seem to be rest, growth and repair. While we're asleep, certain hormones are released, the cells of the body grow and are repaired or renewed, and our brains rest and recover from the rigours of the day's activities. One useful way of trying to understand why we need to sleep is to look at what happens if we don't sleep. Although we may feel physically weak and lethargic when we haven't had enough sleep, it is our brain function that suffers the most. Lack of sleep reduces the brain's capacity for innovative thinking and flexible decision-making; it impairs judgement, affects memory and concentration and shortens your attention span. With continued lack of adequate sleep, the part of the brain that is concerned with memory, speech, planning and sense of time is seriously affected, almost shutting down completely. Apart from the obvious risks to health and safety (which we'll look at in more detail in Chapter 3), lack of sleep can make us clumsy, forgetful, irritable and, of course, sleepy.

What happens to the body while we're asleep?

While we are asleep, the muscles relax, the heart rate is reduced, the breathing becomes slower and deeper, the blood pressure, temperature and pulse rate all fall and the metabolic rate slows down. Also, once we're deeply asleep, the brain releases large quantities of growth hormone, essential for cellular repair and regeneration, bone density and immune function.

Much of the body's growing is done while we're asleep. This is because while we're awake we need the activity of certain hormones to get us through the business of everyday life. Adrenaline, for example, circulates in the body in small quantities all the time we are awake and active. It is needed to stimulate our 'fright or flight' response – the primitive mechanism that allows us to respond instantly to a threatening situation. If you come face to face with a marauding bear or a mad axeman, for example, large quantities of adrenaline are released into the bloodstream. Adrenaline increases your heart rate and blood pressure, and speeds up the rate at which you breathe so that more oxygen is carried to the muscles to enable you either to run for your life or to wrestle the bear or fight the axeman.

Another group of hormones, corticosteroids, are produced while we're awake, and these work closely with adrenaline. These are also 'activity' hormones and are the ones responsible for helping you to get out of bed in the morning, ready to face the new day. Adrenaline and corticosteroids both interfere with the action of growth hormones, so your body is unable to grow and repair itself during the day while these hormones are busy working to help keep you active. Once you are asleep, however, the levels of the activity hormones drop significantly, enabling the growth hormone to stimulate the body's growth and repair function.

Ideally, then, your body should release more growth hormone and less activity hormone at night, and more activity hormone and less growth hormone during the day. If your hormone production is thrown out of kilter, you can end up feeling sluggish and lethargic even after having slept for eight or nine hours. This often happens in people who work night shifts or spilt shifts, people who regularly party late into the night and, of course, insomniacs. What happens is that when you're awake all night your body doesn't produce enough growth hormone, and when you sleep during the day you may produce growth hormone, but its action may be hindered by adrenaline and corticosteroids. As a result, your body is unable to carry out its routine maintenance, and you end up feeling sluggish and generally under par.

The stages of sleep

During the course of a night, our sleep occurs in repeated cycles of around 90–100 minutes. Each cycle is made up of non-rapid eye movement (non-REM) sleep, which is divided into four stages, and rapid eye movement (REM) sleep.

Stage one (light sleep)

This is the period where we shift from wakefulness to almost-sleep. The muscles relax and may twitch slightly, or you may experience a sensation of falling. The blood pressure drops and the heart rate and digestion slow down. Research shows that brain activity changes through the stages, and the electrical signals we call brain waves slow down as sleep deepens. In stage one, the brain emits alpha waves at a rate similar to that of someone who is meditating or under hypnosis – in other words, awake but very relaxed. Someone in stage one sleep, which lasts for up to about ten minutes, can be easily woken.

Stage two (true sleep)

This stage makes up the largest part of our night's sleep. Most noises will not wake someone in stage two sleep, although meaningful noise – someone calling your name or a child crying – is likely to wake you. A mixture of deeper, slower brain waves, called theta and delta waves, is emitted in this stage, during which we are, in effect, unconscious.

Stages three and four (deep sleep)

During stage three, the temperature drops and the heart rate and breathing slow down even more. Delta wave activity increases and we are taken further into deep sleep. Stage four is the stage when we are most deeply asleep and from which it is the most difficult to wake. Delta waves predominate, and if we are woken from this stage we are likely to feel disorientated and groggy for a few minutes. Stages three and four together last for around 30 minutes, after which we go up through the stages again before moving into REM sleep.

REM sleep

REM or 'rapid eye movement' sleep is so called because that's exactly what happens – the eyes dart around so rapidly that the movement can be seen under the eyelids. Also, our breathing and heart rates increase. This kind of sleep is also sometimes called 'paradoxical sleep', because although there is considerable activity going on in the brain, the body is virtually paralysed during this phase. It is mainly during REM sleep that we dream, although we may not remember the dreams, and it is said that the paralysis of the body is nature's way of preventing us from acting out our dreams, thus keeping us safe from harm. The first REM sleep usually occurs about an hour or so after falling asleep. During the course of the night, most people will have between three and five REM episodes, each becoming slightly longer as the night progresses. When we come out of REM sleep, we move back up into stage one and the whole cycle begins again.

It used to be thought that REM sleep was essential to wellbeing and that without it our health, particularly our mental health, would suffer irreparable damage. This is no longer thought to be the case, although studies show that if someone is deprived of REM sleep for more than three days he or she is likely to start hallucinating and having waking dreams.

Why do we dream?

The world of dreams has fascinated humankind for thousands of years, with many theories being developed as to why we dream. Sigmund Freud's fascination with the subject led to his groundbreaking work *The Interpretation of Dreams*, published in 1900. The book marked the beginnings of scientific research into the complexities of the mind; it influenced the way scientists studied the brain because it was the first work to really look at the connection between the mind and the physical lump of tissue contained within the human skull. This helped to develop a deeper understanding of mental illness.

Freud believed that dreams were a means of wish-fulfilment, a way of playing out a repressed sexual or unacceptable desire in disguised form. Later in his life, he conceded that dreams were not always about gratifying hidden wishes – he noted, for example, that some dreams seemed to represent an attempt to come to terms with a past trauma. But he was certain that dreams were made up of both surface and hidden themes of significant importance to the dreamer. He wrote, 'the interpretation of dreams is the royal road to a knowledge of the unconscious activities of the mind'. This was a road along which someone could travel to discover the unconscious desires that were being repressed and were therefore, Freud believed, causing that person's neuroses. It was this theory that led to his development of psychoanalysis, from which many modern psychotherapies have since been developed.

Carl Jung, who worked closely with Freud for a while, disagreed with Freud's theory that dreams were a product of erotic desires that were too outrageous for us to consider consciously. Jung suggested that the purpose of dreaming was to remind us of our wishes, enabling us to realize the things we unconsciously yearn for. Jung believed that dreams were messages from ourselves to ourselves, and that we should pay attention to them for our own benefit. He also developed the concept of the Collective Unconscious – the idea that we are connected to a shared pool of ideas, thoughts and memories that come from the experiences of our ancestors, and indeed from the entire human race. We inherit these primal experiences and memories, which are represented in our dreams by archetypes – images and symbols that are common elements of myths and legends across the globe.

Other theories include the idea that dreams are the brain's way of 'housekeeping' – re-ordering stored information, consolidating learning and memories and discarding information that is no longer useful. It has also been suggested that dreams are a way of making us aware of unresolved problems, or of helping us to find solutions. It may even be that dreaming is a way of keeping us entertained while we sleep!

Even in the twenty-first century, we still cannot be entirely sure about the purpose of dreams, if indeed there is a purpose. However, most people would accept that dreams can be a rich source of creativity – many writers, poets and artists have found inspiration in the form of dreams. It is also true that dreams can be emotionally healing: for example, when one awakes comforted by a dream in which one has been able to spend a little time with a deceased relative, friend or pet.

If you're interested in the content of your dreams, it might be an idea to keep a 'dream diary' by your bed, so that you can jot the dream down while it's fresh in your memory. Often, when you look at the various elements of the dream, you'll find it is simply a melting pot of things that you've seen and heard throughout the day. However, it may be that some parts of the dream represent particular things or have particular meaning for you, and this may become clear over time as you find certain themes recurring.

Dreaming can be a problem if it is contributing to your insomnia – for example, if the dreams cause you to awaken frequently during the night – especially if you then have trouble getting back to sleep. If you suffer distressing dreams or nightmares, you may find you are reluctantly staying awake rather than submitting yourself to unpleasant dreams that cause fear or distress. We all have nightmares now and again, but if this is a persistent problem it's possible that something is bothering you that you may or may not be consciously aware of. If you're not sure what's causing them, keep a record of your distressing dreams. With a written record spanning a few weeks, you may be able to work out what's causing your nightmares. This may be enough to help you to deal with the problem, but it may be worth looking into the possibility of having some counselling to try and help you to understand and deal with whatever it is that's bothering you. (See Chapter 8 for more about nightmares.)

How much sleep do we need?

Most magazine or internet articles about sleep will tell you that the majority of people need around seven to eight hours a night. But we know there are huge variations in people's sleep patterns, with some sleeping only a few hours a night and others needing nine or even ten hours in order to feel refreshed. Margaret Thatcher famously claimed to need just four hours' sleep a night, and most new mothers find they can function reasonably well on little more than that. Dr Chris Idzikowski, director of the Edinburgh Sleep Centre, says, 'The amount of sleep you need is the amount it takes so that you are not tired the next day.' In other words, if you sleep for eight hours a night but are still sleepy the next day, you may need more than that. Similarly, if you only sleep for five hours but wake feeling fine and get through your day's work without feeling unduly tired, then five hours is probably enough for you.

Studies have shown that people who function well on just a few hours a night tend to skip the lighter stages of sleep, slipping straight from waking into deep sleep. This is usually when the activity hormones are at their lowest levels and the level of growth hormone is at its highest, which perhaps explains how these people cope with so little sleep.

Can you train yourself to need less sleep?

While it's true that you can get used to having less sleep, research suggests that the amount of sleep you need doesn't change. One study looked at nuns in a convent whose lifestyle meant that they slept far less than average. The nuns were given special dispensation to take part in the study, which allowed them to sleep for as long as they wished in the mornings. Their sleep quickly moved back to what would be considered a more normal pattern. This suggests that even after years of training, although the nuns' bodies were coping on less sleep, their fundamental sleep needs remained unchanged.

The effects of ageing on sleep

Age is a big factor in what constitutes a normal amount of sleep. For example, the average newborn baby sleeps around 16 hours out of every 24, whereas a four-year-old will probably sleep for around 12 hours. Someone who's 18 or 19 will probably sleep for longer than someone in their forties, and the average 70-year-old is likely to have a better night than someone who's 90. This does not mean that we need less sleep as we get older, only that we tend not to get as much sleep in later life. The amount of REM or paradoxical sleep we have in any one night tends to remain fairly unchanged as we age; what changes is the amount of deep sleep. An elderly person will have roughly the same amount of REM sleep as a much younger person, but may only spend half the amount of time in deep sleep (stages three and four). This is why older people often doze off during the daytime – far from needing less sleep than younger people, they are in fact deprived of essential restorative sleep.

Some myths about sleep

There are a number of myths about sleep. These can lead to unnecessary anxiety and can actually cause sleep difficulties in people who were previously sleeping normally. Some of the most common myths are:

1 *Human beings need eight hours' sleep a night.*
   As we have seen, the amount of sleep needed varies from person to person. For most people, the odd bad night will not cause too many problems, although if you frequently feel sleepy the

following day, it could be that you're not getting enough good quality sleep.

2 *The older you get, the less sleep you need.*
This is not true. Older people need the same amount of sleep, with the same individual variations, as anyone else, though they may suffer more sleep disruption as a result of age-related health or other issues, such as needing to go to the loo more often.

3 *Turning up the car radio will help keep you awake while driving.*
Turning the volume up, opening the window or switching on the air conditioning may all help temporarily, but eventually the brain of a tired driver will block these things out and he or she may fall asleep at the wheel. At the very least, his or her reactions will be affected.

4 *The human body can adjust to night-shift work.*
Although some people may get used to being awake all night and sleeping during the day, we are actually programmed to feel more sleepy during the hours of darkness. Shift work disrupts this programming and shift workers frequently experience sleep disorders as a result. Workers whose shifts vary, switching from day to night and back again within fairly short periods, are particularly at risk of sleep disturbance and a number of associated illnesses.

5 *Snoring is annoying but not harmful.*
Snoring itself is not harmful, but as well causing social and marital problems, it can also indicate the presence of *sleep apnoea,* a potentially life-threatening condition where someone stops breathing during sleep (see p. 51). When you stop breathing your brain automatically wakes you up, usually with a loud snore or snort, so that you start breathing again. You won't remember waking, but this can happen many times during a night's sleep, leaving you sleepy and with slowed reactions the following day. A driver with sleep apnoea is roughly seven times more likely to have a road accident, and driver sleepiness is thought to cause around one in ten road crashes.

6 *If you miss out on sleep, you can catch up by having more the following night.*

If you miss out on a few hours' sleep, the best thing you can do is to try to get back to normal the following night. Lost sleep is lost for good – you can't 'catch up' as such. After several nights of insufficient sleep, you can build up a 'sleep debt', and because you can't 'clear' that debt by having extra-long periods of sleep, the lack of sleep is likely to affect your day-to-day functioning.

7 *If you wake in the night, the best thing you can do is to lie quietly or count sheep until you fall asleep again.*

This is not a good idea unless you're fairly sure you'll drop off again soon. Usually, the more you lie there *trying* to get to sleep, the more difficult it becomes. Instead of tossing and turning, get up and do something: read a boring book, perhaps, or take a warm bath.

8 *If you're sleepy during the day, it means you just need to go to bed earlier.*

This is sometimes the case, but not always. Clearly, if you've stayed up late to watch a film or you've been out to a party and you're sleepy the next day, it's probably because you had a fairly short night. However, if you're sleepy even after a reasonable amount of sleep, it may be that something is preventing you from having refreshing sleep, for example sleep apnoea (see p. 51) or restless legs syndrome (see p. 44). The quality of your sleep is often more important than the quantity.

9 *Teenagers who sleep late are just lazy.*

Growing teenagers need quite a lot of sleep – more than adults, in fact. But having to get up early for school when they've stayed up late socializing, studying or doing part-time work means that few teenagers get the sleep they actually need.

10 *A few drinks before bed will help you sleep.*

It's certainly true that alcohol has a sedative effect and it may indeed cause you to fall asleep more quickly. However, alcohol is likely to disrupt your sleep patterns so that, although you may sleep heavily for the first three or four hours, after that you're more likely to snore and to wake frequently throughout the night. And in the morning, even if you're lucky enough to escape the dreaded hangover, you're unlikely to feel refreshed and may be sluggish and lethargic for at least part of the day.

2

Understanding insomnia

Many people assume that people with 'insomnia' are those who have difficulty falling asleep. In fact, you can fall asleep as soon as you get into bed and still be suffering from insomnia. A more accurate definition of the condition is when someone frequently has inadequate or poor quality sleep due to difficulty falling asleep or staying asleep, waking up too early and not being able to get back to sleep and/or waking up feeling unrefreshed. In order to understand insomnia, we need to look at how the body is 'programmed' to sleep, and what happens when this programming is disrupted.

Circadian rhythms: the body clock

Our bodies are naturally programmed to run on a cycle of roughly 24 hours, set in time with the rising and setting of the sun and determining when we naturally wake and sleep. This cycle or rhythm is known as the circadian rhythm (from the Latin *circa*, meaning 'around', and *diem*, meaning 'day') and is the correct term for what we more often refer to as the 'body clock'. The normal cycle of sleeping and wakefulness can, if disrupted, cause us to have difficulty sleeping. Circadian rhythms are responsible for controlling changes in body temperature, and also for changes in hormone levels in response to daylight. During the early evening, our body temperature is at its highest. It then starts to fall, reaching its lowest level in the early hours of the morning, which is usually when we find it easiest to fall asleep. It then starts to slowly rise again before we wake. In terms of hormones, the onset of darkness stimulates the pineal gland at the centre of the brain to secrete large amounts of melatonin, a hormone that makes us feel drowsy and helps to keep us asleep. Melatonin levels are at their highest during the hours of darkness, peaking at around 3 a.m. When the sun rises, light penetrates the brain via the retina, causing melatonin production to cease and stimulating the release of 'waking' and activity hormones. This is the principle on which dawn or sunrise simulator alarm clocks work. These clocks take the form of a bedside lamp, and instead of waking you with a loud noise, they work by gradually getting brighter, with a type of light very similar to natural daylight. This is a much more gentle way of waking than a blaring alarm clock and can be very useful for people with sleep disorders (see p. 75 for more about light therapy).

If we look at people who work night shifts, we find that no matter how stimulating the activity they're involved in at the time, they are likely to experience a dip in alertness at around 3 a.m., when melatonin levels are high and temperature is low – the best conditions for sleep. Similarly, even if they've worked a long and tiring shift, when they arrive home at around nine in the morning they're likely to feel awake and even refreshed, making it difficult for them to go to sleep when we would expect them to be feeling exhausted.

Ultradian rhythms

While the circadian rhythm controls the 24-hour wake and sleep cycle, the ultradian rhythm is responsible for shorter and more frequent 'mini-cycles' we experience throughout the day and night. These cycles last around 90 minutes and will contain 'peaks' and 'troughs' of alertness. This can explain why you might suddenly feel very sleepy at one point during the day and then feel wide awake half an hour later, even when you've not had any sleep. Some people find that they are more productive when they take a short break every 90 minutes or so than when they work solidly for four hours either side of one long break in the middle of the day. Unfortunately, the current culture of working long hours with few breaks means that even those who know they can achieve more by working to a different pattern from their colleagues are reluctant to take breaks in case they're seen as weak or not 'up to the job'.

Owls and larks

Are you an 'early bird'? Do you leap out of bed at first light, ready to face the day and knowing you'll get loads done if you can get started by eight or nine o'clock? Or are you one of those who lives in dread of the alarm clock, staggering bleary-eyed from the bedroom with a mumbled protest that you 'don't do mornings'? Most of us know whether we feel at our best in the morning or in the evening, but for some people the difference is so extreme that trying to function outside of their natural rhythm makes life very difficult.

Larks tend to get up early, feel wide awake soon after rising and are able to get on with their work or other commitments quite readily. They may feel several dips during the course of the day, the first coming at around 10.30 or 11 a.m. when blood sugar is running low. This is why we tend to take a coffee break around mid-morning. The period just after lunch is another time when larks feel sluggish, with a further low point coming later in the afternoon, by which time many larks are ready for a nap. Larks' alertness continues to decline during the evening and they're usually ready for bed by ten, where they'll doze off fairly quickly, sleeping quite deeply, often until six or seven when they wake easily, raring to go all over again. If the lark has to get up an hour earlier for some reason, it's usually fairly easy for him or her to cope. But larks find it quite difficult to stay up late, even on special occasions.

For owls, on the other hand, an early start would be little short of torture. Owls struggle to wake up and may find it takes them an hour or two to get going in the morning. As the day progresses, however, owls tend to perk up and become increasingly alert, functioning better and better (with the odd dip in alertness, just like the lark) until they reach their peak in the evening. By bedtime – or what most people regard as bedtime – the owl is wide awake and has little chance of going to sleep, so late nights and parties are easy to deal with. If owls have an unusually late night, they just sleep for longer in the morning. Unlike the lark, the owl spends longer periods in the lighter stages of sleep and takes a long time to fall into a deep, refreshing slumber. Often, owls find themselves still in relatively deep sleep when it's time to get up. This can make them feel disoriented, irritable and of course, sleepy.

For self-employed owls who are able to set their own patterns of work and sleep, this may be less of a problem than for those who have to be up early to catch the 7.30 train to the city. However, even if you're lucky enough to be able to organize your life so that you can work all night, you may still find that your sleep pattern causes problems in your social life and relationships. If one partner is sleeping all day, for example, it puts quite a strain on the other partner, who has to keep the kids quiet and leap on the telephone as soon as it rings.

So why do some people have such extreme differences when it comes to their sleep patterns? Recent research suggests there may be a genetic explanation. Scientists have identified a genetic muta-tion, which they have called the 'after-hours gene'. Experiments observing when and how often mice chose to run on an exercise wheel showed that some of the creatures seemed to run on a 27-hour body clock rather than the usual 24-hour cycle. Those mice who displayed the tendency to a 27-hour pattern were found to have the 'after-hours' version of the Fbxl3 gene, one of a family of genes that controls the breakdown of certain proteins within the body cells. The discovery of the after-hours gene could have significant implications in the development of drugs to help people adjust to shift work or jet lag.

Who is most likely to suffer from sleep difficulties?

Most of us will have difficulty sleeping at some point in our lives, so it really is an issue that concerns everyone. But some people are more likely to suffer insomnia than others.

Shift workers

Those who work night shifts are more prone to sleep difficulties because of the disruption to their circadian rhythms. This throws off the timing of the release of various hormones and makes it very difficult for the body to adjust to a sleep and waking pattern that goes against its natural programming. As we have seen, those whom we would term 'night owls' find it slightly easier to cope with night work. However, many jobs that require shift work involve frequent changes from day shifts to night shifts, which means there is never enough time for the body clock to readjust. It takes around a week to ten days for your body to adapt to a new sleep pattern, but many jobs involve irregular shift patterns where employees are asked to work, say, four night shifts, then three days off, then four day shifts. This sort of pattern really throws a proverbial spanner into the mechanism of the body clock and the body never quite gets used to any particular pattern. Even regular night workers experience problems when, in order to fit in with domestic and social life, they try to return to a more 'normal' pattern at weekends. Although some people will find it easier to cope than others, the body clock cannot adjust completely because of the effect of light on the release of hormones. So, even if you manage to get through your night shift without falling asleep, the chances are that when you're trying to sleep during the day, light penetration will send the message to your brain that you should be awake. The brain then changes your hormone levels and body temperature accordingly, making it almost impossible for you to doze off. It may be possible to trick your body clock to a certain extent by using light therapy (see p. 75) and by making sure your daytime sleep environment is as dark as possible (see Chapter 6 for more on improving your sleep environment).

Andy

Andy, 34, has recently changed jobs and is trying to readjust after more than 12 years of shift work.

> My body clock was all over the place when I first left my old job. I worked for a fast-food chain and our shift patterns were quite erratic – I'd be working from 8 a.m. until 4 p.m. one day, then a day off, then 4 p.m. until midnight for a couple of days, then back to 8–4. If I worked until midnight, it would often be 12.30 or 1 a.m. before I'd actually finish, 1.30 by the time I got home and 3.30 or 4 a.m. before I got to sleep. You can't just come home after a busy late shift and fall asleep – your mind is too active. I'd often stay up and have a couple of beers or watch a film before I went to bed – that's what normal people do after a day's work, isn't it? But it started to get so that I couldn't sleep. Often, I'd lie there wide awake until it got light, then I'd doze off eventually and would be unable to get up for work. I was late all the time, and in the

end I was just walking around like a zombie. I thought I'd better leave before they sacked me.

I started a new job six weeks ago. It's still shift work, but it's much more civilized – I work 8 a.m.–4 p.m. or 11 a.m.–7 p.m. I took a couple of weeks off between jobs to try and readjust, but it's really difficult and I'm having a lot of trouble getting to sleep at night. I tried some over-the-counter remedy, and it made me feel quite relaxed but I still didn't go to sleep. I'm now trying light therapy – my wife read an article in a magazine about how you can use these special lamp-alarm clocks to 're-set' your body clock. I've only been using it for about ten days, but I am managing to go to sleep and wake up a little earlier – and I've only been late for work once!

Jet lag

People who frequently travel by air suffer very similar reactions to shift workers in that they may find it difficult to get to sleep or to stay asleep, the result being that they feel sluggish and sleepy during the day. 'Jet lag', as it is popularly known, is caused by crossing into a new time zone faster than the body can adapt. If you cross two or three time zones, the problem becomes even more severe. If jet lag only affects you for a couple of days at either end of the annual family holiday, it may not cause serious problems. However, if you travel frequently for work or family reasons, it can be debilitating. Chapter 5 looks at possible solutions for jet lag.

Women

Studies suggest that insomnia is more common among women than men, and this may be largely due to the effects of certain hormones, as well as to lifestyle issues.

During pregnancy, for example, you're likely to need the loo more often, and as the pregnancy progresses, the pressure of the growing baby on the bladder can wake you up even when you don't need to urinate. Increasing foetal movement may keep you awake, and eventually the change in body shape and the extra weight can make you uncomfortable at night. If we then consider the natural anxieties about the coming birth and the associated lifestyle changes, we can see why pregnancy can cause sleeping difficulties. Unfortunately, things don't tend to improve after the baby is born – at least, not for a while.

If you're a new mum, the chances are you can no longer remember what a good night's sleep is like. Almost all new parents suffer some level of sleep deprivation, but mums tend to miss out on sleep more than dads. This may be because mothers often take the main responsibility for getting up at night, or it may be that breastfeeding prevents them from sleeping for more than a couple of hours at a time. Even when women are no longer what we'd call 'new' mothers, many say that their sleep is generally lighter than before they gave birth because they are constantly on the alert for the sound of a child crying.

Later in life, the menopause and the time leading up to it, known as the peri-menopause, can cause problems for women in terms of sleep. Hot flushes and night sweats caused by hormonal changes can wreak havoc with your sleep. In addition, the menopause can be a time when other stresses and strains come to the fore. The menopause may coincide with 'empty nest syndrome' as children start to leave home, or other lifestyle changes such as reduced working hours or early retirement, relationship difficulties or increased responsibility for elderly parents. You may feel a sense of grief for your lost fertility and also be affected by fears and worries associated with getting older. The menopause can be difficult both physically and emotionally, and it's not uncommon for women to report quite serious sleep disturbances around this time. Physical symptoms such as hot flushes may be relieved by HRT, or by natural alternatives such as black cohosh or red clover. Emotional problems are more trouble-some to solve, but talking them over with a counsellor may help.

Even without the hormone connection, for many women a busy lifestyle alone is enough to disrupt sleep, especially for those who are working wives and mothers. Survey after survey tells us that, even in the twenty-first century, it is women who do the vast majority of housework, laundry, shopping, cooking, childcare and domestic accounting. If a woman also does paid work, the domestic chores can stretch well into late evening, and it is not uncommon for a woman still to be making packed lunches, ironing shirts or dealing with household admin long after the rest of the family has retired. Without the normal unwinding period between work and bed, many women find it difficult to relax and fall asleep for some time after getting into bed.

Older people

The fact that sleep difficulties are common in older people has led to the popular myth that we need less sleep as we age. In fact, one of the reasons older people often doze during the day is because they do not have sufficient sleep at night. We know that sleep tends to be lighter as we get older but there are a number of other factors that may be involved. Some health problems can affect your ability to sleep well, and Chapter 5 looks at a few of the more common conditions. A change in lifestyle can also make sleep more elusive for the older person. Moderate exercise is known to have a beneficial effect on sleep, for example, but we tend to take less exercise as we age. A recent study in people over 65 found that going for a brisk 30–40 minute walk four times a week helped them to fall asleep more quickly and stay asleep for longer. The exercise also seemed to improve the quality of their sleep, making them feel more refreshed on waking. Elderly people who go to bed earlier and earlier will, not surprisingly, find that they wake earlier. This may cause a slight change in the setting of the body clock in the same way that teenagers often go to bed later and later, causing a similar change but in reverse. If you are living in a retirement or nursing home, you may find that the daily routine there makes it difficult for you to follow your normal sleep pattern. This could be because residents are encouraged to go to bed earlier than they might wish to, or it may simply be that there is a certain amount of environmental disturbance such as light or noise from overnight staff, or from other residents.

Social and psychological factors such as loneliness, stress and depression are fairly common in older people, and this can affect your sleep in old age. It should also be borne in mind that lack of restorative sleep over a significant length of time can actually cause depression, so it's important to try and ascertain whether it's depression that's causing your insomnia or the other way round. See Chapter 4 for more about how depression and related conditions may affect sleep.

The overall amount of sleep is probably more important than the length of time you stay asleep overnight. So if, for example, you used to sleep for eight hours a night when you were younger and now find you only sleep for six, it is quite normal for you to take a couple of hour-long naps during the day. If this pattern of sleeping doesn't cause you too many problems, don't worry about it. If, however, you find that you're still feeling unrefreshed or that you're often sleepy and lethargic during the day, you may need some help to identify and treat the reason, so talk to your doctor about this. You may also find Chapters 4 and 5 helpful in terms of identifying particular conditions and solutions, and for some self-help suggestions have a look at Chapter 6.

3

Do you have insomnia?

As we have seen, many people assume that unless you lie awake for hours, tossing and turning in your tangled bed, you're not an insomniac. But insomnia doesn't just mean that you have difficulty getting to sleep at night; you may be asleep within five minutes of going to bed but still have insomnia. You probably have insomnia if you frequently experience wakefulness or disturbed sleep *and* tiredness is affecting your mood and/or your normal functioning the following day: for example, if you feel sleepy, fatigued and irritable, or if your concentration, memory and ability to work is reduced because of your tiredness. Let's look at the various ways it can affect you.

Difficulty getting to sleep

If you're frequently still awake 20 minutes or more after settling down and closing your eyes, this will be classed as insomnia. There may be several factors contributing to your inability to drop off. For example:

Weekend sleep disruption

Here's the scenario. You have a takeaway on Friday night (after all, it *is* Friday) and maybe a few drinks (after all, you've worked hard all week) and you stay up later than usual. The alcohol makes you go to sleep quite quickly, but you have a disturbed night because it also makes you get up to go to the loo; and your stomach's a little uncomfortable because of the curry you had at 9.30 p.m. Having gone to bed later than usual and had disturbed sleep, you find it hard to get up on Saturday morning. You may even have a hangover, making it that much more difficult to drag yourself out of bed. Eventually you get up, revive yourself to a certain extent with tea and toast and get on with your day. By 4 p.m., though, you're feeling the ill-effects of your late night so, as it's the weekend, you decide to have a nap to perk yourself up ready for the evening – after all, it *is* Saturday night. You hadn't realized quite how tired you were and you sleep for an hour and a half; you must have needed it, and you feel so much better. So then you go out for the evening, or you have friends over, or you stay up and watch the late film, probably with a couple of glasses of wine, because after all, it *is* Saturday night. You end up going to bed much later than usual, because you don't feel tired (having had a long nap in the afternoon) and you're having a nice time and anyway, it *is* Saturday night. By the time you crawl from your bed on Sunday, the morning has almost gone. You get on with your day but you're very aware that it's Monday tomorrow and you need to be up at 6.45, so you'd better have an early night. But of course, you can't sleep. Typical!

Sound familiar? Tempting though it is to stay up late when you don't have commitments the following day, this can cause real problems, especially if you're prone to sleeplessness. It really is better to try and stick to roughly the same bedtime every night, going to bed no more than an hour later than usual at weekends.

Busy bedrooms

An associated problem is that if, after a couple of late nights, you go to bed before you're really tired, it's tempting to pick up a book, switch the television on or even catch up on paperwork until you feel drowsy enough to turn the light off. The result is that you start to associate the bedroom with activities other than sleep; this means that when you go to bed, your brain no longer expects to sleep, and so it will take longer to wind down. Sleep experts tell us that apart from sleeping, the only thing that should happen in bed is sex.

Underlying worries

It is very common for people who are stressed or worried about something to have difficulty falling asleep. We all know how hard it is to mentally 'switch off' when something is worrying us. This may be a short-lived nuisance if, for example, there is a particular event such as an exam or job interview coming up that you feel anxious about, in which case sleep usually improves once the event has passed. For some people, it is an ongoing situation that keeps them awake – debt, for example, relationship difficulties or problems at work. Major life-events, whether they're distressing events such as bereavement or divorce, or happy, exciting things like moving house, being promoted or getting married, can also disturb your normal sleep pattern. If you are experiencing these sorts of difficulties the advice in Chapter 6 might be useful, but you will need to address any underlying problems as well, and Chapter 4 might offer some useful suggestions.

Other factors

Other causes of being unable to fall asleep include body-clock disturbances caused by jet lag or shift work, environmental problems such as noise and temperature, and consuming too much caffeine, especially in the evening. Studies show that even in people who normally sleep well, a cup of coffee late at night can delay the onset of sleep by around 40 minutes. Caffeine doesn't affect everyone in the same way, but it's easy enough to tell if it's keeping you awake; if so, try not to drink too much tea and coffee during the day and avoid it altogether for a couple of hours before bedtime. Be aware also that over-the-counter medicines, including some headache tablets, may contain caffeine.

Waking during the night

For some people, the problem is not so much getting to sleep as staying asleep. All the factors that prevent someone from going to sleep can also cause them to wake during the night; but there are other common causes, such as alcohol consumption – one of the main causes of night waking. This is partly because alcohol is a diuretic, which means it increases urination and causes dehydration, so apart from having to get up to go to the loo, you're also likely to wake up because you're thirsty. People who are going through alcohol withdrawal are also prone to night waking, as are those who are withdrawing from certain drugs. Other causes include illness, pain or discomfort, conditions such as sleep apnoea (see p. 51) or restless legs syndrome (see p. 44) and, for women who are going through the menopause, hot flushes or night sweats.

Early morning waking

Waking up early and being unable to go back to sleep can also be caused by the things already mentioned. In addition, depression and alcoholism may be factors, as may dependency on sleeping pills. This can happen when tolerance to the drug increases so that larger and larger doses are needed to achieve the same result. Sleeping pills are discussed in more depth in Chapter 7. Another common cause of early waking is simply going to bed too early. As we have seen, we're constantly told that a 'normal' night's sleep is between seven and eight hours, and so if we wake after six hours, we may think we haven't had enough sleep. In fact, if you frequently wake after six hours, it may just be that you don't need any more sleep than that. If you can't find another reason for your early waking, try staying up a little later; then, assuming you sleep later in accordance with the later bedtime, get up when you wake and see how you feel.

Poor quality sleep

This is when, having gone to sleep at your normal time, you wake feeling unrefreshed, as though you've been up half the night. You may feel sleepy, sluggish, irritable and generally unwell. It is quite likely that your reactions will be slower and your performance at work may be affected. This can happen when you're getting plenty of light sleep but are not spending enough time in the deeper, more refreshing levels of sleep. This is common in the elderly, and explains why older people often feel the need to take regular naps during the day. Alcohol, while it may help you to doze off, can prevent you from slipping into deep sleep. In fact, studies on the sleep patterns of alcoholics show that their sleep is very similar to that of elderly people, with longer periods of light sleep and little or no deep sleep. Poor quality sleep may also be a problem if you suffer from sleep apnoea (see p. 51), a condition that causes you to wake many times over the course of a night. Each period of wakefulness is so brief that you probably won't remember it, but again it means that deep, restorative sleep remains elusive.

Conditioned insomnia

Sometimes, the experience of insomnia can itself become a cause, even when the original cause no longer applies. For example, somebody suffering from insomnia due to a period of financial insecurity may spend long sleepless nights feeling anxious about mounting debts. After a while, he or she begins to associate going to bed with anxiety and distress, and this 'conditions' the person to expect a sleepless night. This can sometimes start in childhood when children have been sent to bed for being naughty. They come to associate going to bed with anger and punishment, or with their own feelings of guilt or even fear. Children who are sent to bed far too early, even if not in anger, may become used to lying awake for a long time. They become conditioned to expect wakefulness, and this may continue into adulthood. This type of insomnia may also affect people who have been told that they need seven or eight hours a night in order to function. They worry that they won't get enough sleep, and in the end the worry about whether they'll be able to sleep actually ends up keeping them awake! People who suffer conditioned insomnia often find they feel pleasantly sleepy until they actually get into bed, and that's when the problem starts. They may find that they sleep well on holiday or when staying with friends – a different bedroom often does the trick.

Sarah

Sarah is 48 and has suffered from insomnia on and off for most of her life. She thinks she may have conditioned herself to stay awake as a child.

> I've had trouble sleeping for as long as I can remember. As a child, I had to pretend I was asleep when Santa came because my parents told me he wouldn't come while I was still awake. My mum tells me that when I was very little, I used to stay awake deliberately because I wanted to know where I went when I went to sleep! Maybe that was what started it, but the difficulty getting to sleep lasted well into my teens – I remember lying awake watching the lights in the high-rise block opposite go off one by one until I felt I was the only person in the world who was still awake.
>
> When I had children, I would collapse into bed exhausted and fall asleep quickly, only to be woken through the night by a crying child.

Now the kids have grown up, I still wake several times a night, which I think is a hangover from those early days of parenthood. Mostly, I go back to sleep, but for some reason if I wake at 4 a.m. I'm usually awake for at least an hour, sometimes two. I think it may have become a conditioned response – I look at the clock and think, *oh no, now I won't be able to get back to sleep.* I've found the best thing to do is to just get up and read for a while. If I do this, I usually feel sleepy again around 5.30 so I go back to bed. If it happens a few nights in succession, I take a herbal remedy called Sedonium (see p. 76) for a couple of nights. That seems to break the habit. Insomnia can be very unpleasant, even if you're lucky enough to be able to take a nap during the day. When it's 4 a.m., your partner is sleeping peacefully, the street outside is deserted and silent and there are no lights on in any of the houses, it's no fun being the only one awake.

What are the consequences?

Most of us can cope with the odd bad night. We can even cope with slightly longer periods of disturbed sleep if we know it is a temporary situation, but chronic or recurrent insomnia can have a devastating effect on your daily life and should be addressed just as you would address any other health problem. In fact, there is increasing evidence to suggest there may be a link between insufficient sleep and a higher risk of major illnesses such as heart disease, diabetes, some cancers and obesity. There also seems to be a greater prevalence of emotional and psychological problems, including depression. The exact reasons are not yet clear, and research continues. What is clear, however, is the significantly increased risk of accident or error as a result of insufficient or poor quality sleep.

Daytime tiredness and sleepiness

Sleep difficulties can cause daytime tiredness and sleepiness. Tiredness is slightly different to sleepiness in that you're also likely to lack energy and motivation as well as feeling generally lethargic and fatigued. Sleepiness is an abnormal and prolonged feeling of drowsiness, often with a tendency to actually fall asleep at inappropriate times, even while driving. Both are common symptoms of sleep disorders although they can have other causes, such as depression or medical conditions such as anaemia or hypothyroidism, and as a side effect of certain medications.

People who are fatigued are likely to be less efficient, their reactions may be slow and their decision-making may be affected. There has long been concern about the quality of decision-making by junior doctors who have been working for long hours, often without a break, in stressful and demanding situations. Until fairly recently, it was not uncommon for a junior doctor to work for more than 80 hours a week. The introduction of the European Working Time Directive in 2004 means junior doctors should not have to work more than 58 hours a week. This should be reduced to 48 hours by 2009. However, according to the Royal College of Physicians, poorly designed rotas mean that almost half of doctors end up working seven 13-hour shifts in a row, resulting in a 91-hour week! Another study from New Zealand found that two-thirds of junior doctors admitted to having made a mistake through tiredness, with four out of ten having done so in the previous six months. It has been suggested that sleep deprivation has been a significant factor in a number of cases where tired doctors have made serious or even fatal errors in patient care.

Risk of accidents

The likelihood of accidents and injuries is increased because sleep deprivation affects most components of performance in some way. Excessive sleepiness is associated with poor memory and concentration, short attention span, lack of co-ordination and a reduced ability to process information. As a result, the risk of an accident or a serious error of judgement is significantly increased. In some cases, sleep-deprived people may actually fall asleep while at work or while driving.

Studies suggest that just 18 hours without sleep can cause a decrease in performance equivalent to having a blood alcohol level of 0.05 per cent – roughly what you'd expect after drinking two small glasses of wine. After 21 hours of wakefulness, it's equivalent to 0.08 per cent – the current legal drink-driving limit in the UK. In practice, this level of impairment could mean that someone's ability to fully understand or respond to an unexpected situation is severely reduced. This particularly affects drivers. According to the Royal Society for the Prevention of Accidents, driver fatigue is thought to be responsible for thousands of road traffic accidents each year. Research carried out for the Sleep Research Centre at Loughborough University found that 20 per cent of accidents on monotonous roads, such as motorways, are fatigue-related. Similarly, a survey carried out by the Royal College of Physicians of over 1,600 of that notoriously sleep-deprived bunch, junior doctors, found that one in six had had a road accident while travelling to or from work in 2004–5. The greatest risk was found to be when the doctors were returning from a night shift.

Fatigue-related traffic accidents tend to be more serious, probably because the driver is unable to brake or take any avoiding action before the collision. Drivers who are most at risk of falling asleep while driving tend to be shift workers, truck drivers, young male drivers and drivers of company cars. It's worth bearing in mind that if you decide to drive while tired, it is not only yourself and any passengers you are putting at risk: you are also risking the lives of pedestrians and other drivers. It is not currently a specific offence to drive when tired, but there have been a number of successful convictions of drivers who fell asleep at the wheel. These include that of the driver of the Land Rover that left the road and came to rest on a railway line, causing the Selby rail disaster in 2001.

To reduce the risk of accidents on the road:

- Before starting a long journey, make sure you're sufficiently well rested and that you haven't taken any medication that may cause drowsiness.
- Plan your journey to include regular rest breaks – at least 15 minutes every two hours. If necessary, plan an overnight stop.
- Avoid setting out on a long drive at the end of a full working day (or night!).
- Avoid driving at the time when you would normally be falling asleep.
- Avoid driving between 2 a.m. and 6 a.m., and be extra careful when driving between 2 p.m. and 4 p.m., as these are the times when fatigue-related accidents are most common.
- If you feel sleepy during a journey, stop somewhere safe as soon

as possible, drink something containing caffeine and then take a 15 minute nap (the caffeine will take about 15 minutes to kick in) before resuming your journey.

Tiredness also increases the risk of accidents in the home and workplace for the same reasons, i.e. poor concentration, memory lapses, lack of co-ordination, slowed reaction times and a reduced ability to process information. If you're suffering from the effects of sleep deprivation, whether you're up a ladder cleaning out the gutters, in the kitchen frying chips or in front of a computer screen at Air Traffic Control, you could be risking serious injury or death to yourself and others. In fact, it has been suggested that sleep deprivation among shift workers was a contributory factor in a number of international disasters, such as the 1989 Exxon oil spill and the nuclear accidents at Three Mile Island in 1979 and Chernobyl in 1986.

Relationship difficulties

If you suffer persistent sleep difficulties, the chances are you will notice some impact on your relationship with your partner or other family members. Being aware of the potential problems may help, especially if you can discuss these with those close to you so that at least they know what to expect. If they understand the sort of problems that can occur and why, they'll be more likely to be supportive in your attempts to improve the quality of your sleep. In addition, if there is a strain on your relationship with your partner, there will also be a strain on your sex life, which is a shame because sex is the one activity you can do in bed that will actually help you to sleep!

One of the most common problems for the insomniac is lying awake for long periods, wanting to get up and listen to music or have a bath but feeling you can't because you might wake your partner. This can lead to resentment. You may also find that you resent the very fact that your partner is able to sleep while you lie there in the dark for hours, bored stiff and desperate for a break from your conscious mind. Tension can also arise if sleeplessness affects your mood – which it's likely to, let's face it – or if fatigue prevents you from, for example, doing your usual share of the daily chores or taking part in normal family activities.

Even more difficult to cope with is a partner who doesn't believe you have insomnia: '... *but you were asleep as soon as your head hit the pillow'*. Or one who doesn't understand that it is a serious condition and trivializes your tiredness: *'A few bad nights won't hurt you. Just have a cup of coffee and get with it – that's what I always do!'* Unfortunately, people who've never experienced real sleep difficulties don't realize just how debilitating the tiredness that accumulates over time can be, perhaps confusing it with the slightly slow feeling they have after the odd late night. Also, if your partner has slept soundly all night, he or she will assume you have too, especially if you happened to be asleep at the one point when your partner got up to use the loo. This can also lead to the assumption that you're exaggerating your sleeplessness – not that it matters how long you were awake; what matters is how you feel the next day. Someone with sleep apnoea, for example (see p. 51), may appear to sleep quite well, but in fact the condition causes them to wake many times, albeit briefly, leading to a serious risk of fatigue the following day.

Work and social life

These areas of your life are also likely to be affected by your insomnia. If the condition persists, you will often feel below par and may even be irritable with friends and colleagues. Tiredness tends to affect your energy and motivation, which will affect your performance at work. Impaired concentration and decision-making may result in errors, possibly causing conflict with colleagues or with your employer. Your condition may even cost you a valuable promotion, either because you are consistently under-performing or because you're aware that you simply could not cope with the extra responsibility. Your social life may also suffer – when you're feeling fatigued, you probably won't feel like partying, and even popping round to a friend's for a drink or a cup of coffee may seem like too much effort. On other occasions, perhaps, you'll make the effort, only to find that you can barely keep your eyes open and your friends think you're being moody or distant.

How bad is your own insomnia?

If you're not sure just how badly your insomnia is affecting you (perhaps because you're too tired to even think about it!) it may be worth using the Epworth Sleepiness Scale (ESS) to assess the situation. The scale was devised by Dr Murray Johns in Australia and published in 1991, and is now widely used by clinicians all over the world. The scale asks you to rate the likelihood of you dozing off in a number of situations. Even if you haven't been in those situations recently, try to work out how they would have affected you. Use the following scale to choose the most appropriate number of each situation:

0 = Would never doze
1 = Slight chance of dozing
2 = Moderate chance of dozing
3 = High chance of dozing

Situation	Chance of dozing
Sitting and reading	0 1 2 3
Watching television	0 1 2 3
Sitting inactive in a public place (e.g. a theatre)	0 1 2 3
Being a car passenger for an hour without a break	0 1 2 3
Lying down to rest in the afternoon	0 1 2 3
Sitting and talking to someone	0 1 2 3
Sitting quietly after lunch without alcohol	0 1 2 3
In a car, while stopped for a few minutes in traffic	0 1 2 3

Now add up your score:

A score of less than 8 suggests normal sleep function
8–10 = Mild sleepiness
11–15 = Moderate sleepiness
16–20 = Severe sleepiness
21–24 = Excessive sleepiness

Anything more than mild sleepiness indicates some level of sleep disturbance, so you should address this straight away. If your sleepiness is severe or excessive, you should see your doctor without delay.

What can be done?

You will be in little doubt by now that insomnia can be a serious and debilitating condition; whether you're suffering from lack of sleep or poor quality sleep, your health, job, relationship, friendships and even your life can be at risk. Fortunately, there is a great deal that can be done to improve the situation, and the rest of the book will concentrate on identifying possible steps you can take to solve or significantly reduce the severity of the problem.

4

Possible causes (psychological) and solutions

As we have seen, insomnia can have physical, psychological or environmental causes, and often there will be a combination of two or even all three. Just as there is rarely one single cause, there is rarely a single solution, so the best way to approach it is to deal with each component that affects you in the best way you can. This may mean flicking back and forth through the chapters in order to come up with an appropriate insomnia-busting 'package' that fits your individual circumstances. In this chapter, we'll look specifically at psychological factors.

Stress

When we experience stress, the body's 'stress response' kicks in. This involves the release of the hormones adrenaline and cortisol, which are responsible for increasing blood sugar, raising blood pressure and speeding up the heart rate (among other things), to prepare your body for 'fight or flight'. We become more mentally alert and physically more capable of the extra speed and strength we need to escape the perceived threat, whether it's a marauding grizzly bear or a thug in a dark alley with a baseball bat. In the short term, this is a perfectly designed essential response that has helped our species survive.

Unfortunately, stress can also occur when we feel out of control of a situation and unable to cope with the demands placed on us by a demanding job, financial problems or ill health, or of major events such as divorce, bereavement, moving house, children leaving home and so on. The result is that we experience the changes caused by stress for much longer periods than would be necessary for the immediate, intense period of activity required

33

for 'fight or flight'. Prolonged high blood pressure, increased heart rate and raised blood-sugar levels are associated with a number of health problems including heart disease and diabetes. Raised levels of cortisol can affect the immune system as well as affecting your blood pressure, and all that unused adrenaline building up in your system, apart from interfering with your normal sleep–wake patterns, also causes tension in your muscles. When we consider these changes together with the worries or traumatic events that triggered them, it's not surprising that stress can keep us awake!

Not all stress is bad, of course. Changing jobs or even going on holiday can be stressful, but these are also situations that we can find enjoyable. This may be partly due to subjectivity – one person may enjoy sitting exams while another will dread them – but it may also be due to the fact that 'bad' stress – relationship difficulties, illness, financial problems and so on – can make the so-called 'good' stress hard to handle. Whatever the causes, it's clear that stress can affect your ability to sleep, so the first thing to do is learn to recognize the symptoms. Stress affects different people in different ways, but some common symptoms are:

• Sleep disturbances
• Extreme tiredness and lack of energy
• Forgetfulness, inability to concentrate
• Feeling sweaty or shivery
• Panic attacks
• Nausea or 'butterflies' in the stomach
• Headaches or other unexplained aches and pains
• Palpitations
• Dry mouth
• Loss of appetite – for food, sex or fun
• Irritability
• Tearfulness
• Feeling unable to cope.

If you're experiencing five or more of these symptoms, you may be suffering from stress and should take action now. First, you need to try to identify what's causing the stress:

• Relationships – difficulties in relationships with your partner, children, friends, parents, colleagues or even neighbours can take their toll.

- Work – having a heavy workload, feeling undervalued and workplace bullying can all be causes of stress at work. Also, work may be the place where the symptoms of stress become most noticeable, especially when you're also suffering from lack of sleep, and can result in poor performance, lack of concentration and inability to make decisions.
- Financial difficulties – struggling to pay the mortgage or clear rapidly building debts can cause severe stress.
- Ill health – whether it's your own, your partner's or that of a child or parent, illness can be extremely stressful, even if it's not serious or life-threatening. Having to take time off work to care for a sick child or relative, for example, can cause you to worry about the effect on your career.
- Major life-events – changing jobs, marriage, childbirth, retirement, moving house, divorce, children leaving home, bereavement, and so on, can all be stressful.

Obviously there are some things we can't change, but once you've identified the possible cause of your stress, try to find ways of improving the situation. For example, if your workload is too heavy, can you delegate? Can you discuss the situation with your boss? Are there issues at work that could be tackled by your union? If you're having relationship difficulties, can you talk to your partner to try and resolve things? Might it be worth getting some outside help from an organization such as Relate (see p. 110)? If you're worried about debt, could you get financial advice from an organization such as your local Citizens Advice Bureau (see p. 108) or the National Debtline (see p. 110)? If there's nothing you can do to reduce the source of your stress, there are steps you can take to help you cope with it.

First aid for stress

You're at work with a thousand and one things to do, but the phone keeps ringing and your boss is in a bad mood. You're feeling increasingly 'wound up' and if anyone tells you to 'just relax', you won't be responsible for your actions. Sound familiar? When we're stressed, we tend to breathe shallowly, tension builds in our muscles and our shoulders become stiff and high – the feeling that your shoulders are up to your ears. Although meditation and relaxation exercises can be valuable tools to cope with stress, it's not always possible to find a convenient time and place to do them, so sometimes a quick fix is what's needed. This is a useful 'instant' relaxation exercise you can do at any time of day. It only takes a few seconds; you can do it anywhere. Stop whatever you're doing and hunch your shoulders right up. Take a breath in, then very slowly, like a long, deep sigh, let the breath out and at the same time let your shoulders drop down as far as they'll go. Repeat this a couple of times, perhaps visualizing a favourite flower while you do so. Try to keep your shoulders loose and low. Do this as many times through the day as you need to.

Look after your body

The better shape your body is in, the better it is able to cope with the effects of stress. Take a little gentle exercise each day, eat as healthily as possible, cut down on alcohol and if you haven't already done so, give up smoking. Smokers often say they can't give up while they're stressed because a cigarette relieves stress. In fact, smoking a cigarette has the opposite effect: it actually increases the symptoms of stress, and the illusion of stress relief comes from the temporary satisfying of a nicotine craving triggered by the previous cigarette. If you think you'll find it difficult to stop on your own, talk to your doctor. Many doctors' surgeries now have 'quit clinics' that will help smokers find the method of giving up that best suits them. This may be in the form of anti-smoking medication or nicotine replacement therapy, and is often available on prescription.

Rest and relaxation

If you're suffering from stress you're probably not very good at this, and if you're feeling pressured by work or other commitments you're quite likely to say you haven't time for rest and relaxation. But it's essential to allow your body and mind to recharge and recover when you're experiencing stress. Several studies have shown that people who take breaks and know how to 'switch off' are able to achieve as much, and often more, than those who never stop. If it's practical, joining a yoga, meditation or relaxation class may help. If this isn't possible, the exercises in Chapter 6 may be useful (see p. 71). Book a relaxing massage if funds allow, or if you don't fancy that, at least factor in some time every day for a relaxing activity that you enjoy. It may be seeing friends, reading or just listening to music, but make sure it's time spent unwinding – listening to music while you're putting up shelves or doing the ironing doesn't count!

Stress management courses

If you find that there aren't enough hours in the day, as if you're trying to run up the 'down' escalator all the time or you simply don't know where to start in dealing with all your commitments, you may need professional help in managing your stress. Stress management classes may include time management, relaxation and meditation techniques and assertiveness training – with valuable advice on how to say 'no'. Classes may also help you to learn how to handle different types of stress, and how to manage attitudes and behaviours that create or increase stress. For details of courses near you, contact the International Stress Management Association (see p. 109).

Depression

We all feel low sometimes, and lack of sleep, especially if it's affecting your work and personal life, can be at least partially responsible. But there is a huge difference between feeling a bit down and being clinically depressed. If your mood never or rarely lightens, and if you find that you're feeling sad, bleak or hopeless for longer than a few days, you may have depression. It's important to recognize that depression is a potentially life-threatening illness and should be taken seriously. It can affect your ability to deal with your insomnia and your health in general. For example, if you have depression, you're less likely to take physical exercise and more likely to smoke or to drink too much alcohol, all of which makes good quality sleep more elusive. The manifestation of the illness varies from person to person, but these are some of the signs to look out for:

- Inability to fall asleep or early morning wakening
- Lack of energy, fatigue

- Slowed thinking, speech and/or movements
- Inability to concentrate
- Persistent low mood, often worse in the mornings
- Tearfulness
- Feeling unable to experience pleasure or enjoyment
- Loss of interest in social and work activities
- Loss of libido
- Reduced or increased appetite
- Anxiety, panic attacks
- Feelings of worthlessness and hopelessness
- Being able to only see the negative side of things
- Suicidal thoughts.

Note: Depression may also cause someone to sleep for excessively long periods. This is called hypersomnia.

You will notice that some of these symptoms are similar to those of stress (see p. 33), and indeed the two conditions are often closely linked, although they are not the same thing. Stress can be a major cause of depression, although not everyone who is stressed will suffer from depression, and not everyone with depression will have experienced stress. You don't need to have all of these symptoms to be suffering from depression, and indeed some of them – lack of energy and fatigue, for example, or inability to concentrate – are likely to be at least partly due to sleep deprivation. But if you are experiencing some of the other symptoms as well, and if you cannot seem to feel happy or optimistic even when you're not feeling exhausted, you may be depressed. If you're depressed, the chemicals in your brain that govern your mood make it impossible for you to simply 'cheer up'. In fact, telling someone with depression to cheer up or pull him or herself together is like telling someone with a broken leg to go for a run.

What can be done?

The most important thing to remember is that while depression may be a normal result of prolonged sleep deprivation, this does not mean it will go away by itself, so do talk to your doctor. Depression is a serious illness that requires treatment; the good news is that it can be successfully treated in the majority of cases. Your doctor may suggest medication, counselling, cognitive behaviour therapy or a combination of these. Treatment may take several months or even a year or more, and if you're treated with antidepressants it's important to follow the instructions carefully, continuing to take them for at least six months after you last had symptoms, and to gradually reduce the dose rather than just stopping. If taken properly and correctly monitored, antidepressants are a very effective and safe way of treating depression, particularly when used in conjunction with counselling or therapy to address the possible causes. If you choose to find your own therapist, contact the British Association of Counselling and Psychotherapy (BACP) to find a therapist near you (see p. 107).

There may also be things you can do to help improve your mood, such as taking regular exercise, eating or avoiding certain foods, and learning how to change your pattern of negative thinking. There are a number of excellent self-help books that may also be useful; a 'books-on-prescription' scheme launched in Devon in 2004 was so successful that the scheme is now being used in other areas across the country, so you may not even have to buy them. Your doctor will be able to tell you whether the scheme operates in your area, and if so the books should be available at your local library.

Note: There are some herbal preparations that are recommended for mild to moderate depression, but you should not take these without checking with your doctor. St John's Wort, for example, while being an effective and gentle treatment for depression, may affect the action of some medicines, including the contraceptive pill.

Anxiety

Anxiety often goes hand in hand with depression, but it's not the same thing. You can feel sad, bleak and hopeless without necessarily feeling anxious. Anxiety is when you find you can't stop worrying or feeling apprehensive about things. It's natural to worry about ongoing problems or forthcoming difficult situations – it's how we work out what we're going to do to resolve them – but if you do this when you're trying to go to sleep, you will be unable to wind down sufficiently to drop off. It's tempting to avoid thinking about unpleasant things, and during the day, when you're at work or busy dealing with family or domestic responsibilities, it's fairly easy to put your worries to the back of your mind. But if you continually put off thinking about your worries during the day, they are likely to creep back into your mind at night when there's nothing else to distract you. As a result, you may find yourself feeling anxious, unable to put your concerns out of your mind and therefore unable to sleep.

What can you do?

Try to make a conscious effort to think and talk about your concerns during the day, even if this is difficult. By thinking about the problem, talking it over with your partner or a friend and perhaps writing it down, you may be able to find possible solutions. If you're worried about something happening, it may help to plan what you will do if it does. So if, for example, you're worried you might lose your job, make a plan for what you'll do if this happens. This might include things like: *update my CV, telephone employment agencies, find out about benefits, ask the mortgage company if I can reduce the payments for a while.* Making plans will not prevent the worst from happening, but at least you'll know what to do if it does. Having put a well-thought-out plan in place during the day, or even having simply faced your concerns, you'll find it easier to switch off at night. If whatever it is that's causing you to feel anxious is just too much to deal with, it may be that some counselling would help. Talk to your doctor about this, or contact the British Association of Counselling and Psychotherapy (BACP) (see p. 107).

Note: While stress, anxiety and depression are all common factors in insomnia, these conditions can also occur as a result of it. Whether the conditions are the cause or the consequence, the suggestions for treatment and self-help offered here apply equally.

Insomnia following bereavement

Bereavement is one of the most common causes of insomnia, and may trigger the condition even in those who have never experienced it before. The death of someone close to us – a parent, partner, child or friend – can be devastating, but it is something we will all experience at some time, becoming more likely as we get older. It also, of course, forces us to face our own mortality.

Grief affects people differently. When someone you love dies, you may go through a whole range of emotions from sadness, loneliness, despair and longing to fear, anger, resentment and even guilt. Whether or not the death was expected, you may feel a sense of shock that it has actually happened. Or you may be completely numb, as though you can't really feel anything at all. These reactions are all normal; sadly, the bereaved person may not realize this because, thanks to the fact that this most fundamental truth of human existence is still a taboo subject in Western society, we are prevented from openly discussing it. People seem to be embarrassed by grief, and while they may secretly long to offer comfort, their embarrassment makes them reticent. Widows often talk of a double loss: the death of their partner and the loss of former friends who appear to shun them, crossing the road to avoid them rather than offering the longed-for condolences.

Bereavement can be a trigger for all types of insomnia – difficulty falling asleep, frequent night waking, early morning waking and poor quality sleep. If you've lost your partner, you will probably be affected by the fact that, after years of sharing a bed or at least a room with someone else, you're suddenly sleeping alone. This is another factor that can affect your sleep patterns in addition to the emotional distress caused by bereavement. Even though it is perfectly understandable for a bereaved person to have difficulty sleeping, this doesn't mean it will settle down on its own and can therefore be ignored. If you've just lost someone you love, you're more vulnerable to depression and anxiety, and also to various physical illnesses. If the insomnia goes untreated, it can be a factor in more long-term depression and, as we've already seen, depression can itself be a factor in insomnia. So as you can see, it's very easy to quickly fall into a 'vicious circle' situation.

Coping with bereavement-related insomnia

If your insomnia has come on very suddenly after bereavement, it's important to address it quickly to try to prevent it from becoming a serious long-term condition. Chapter 6 contains lots of advice on steps you can take to improve your sleep, but if these have little or no effect, do talk to your doctor about your sleep difficulties. Bereaved people often feel that, because sleeplessness is to be expected, there's no point in mentioning it to their doctor. In fact, your doctor should be keen to address your sleep difficulties because in addition to improving your overall health, you're likely to be better able to cope with the pain of bereavement if you can at least get a reasonable night's sleep.

If your insomnia continues for more than a few nights, it's likely that your whole sleep pattern will change as you become used to lying awake for long periods. Your doctor may suggest a short course of sleeping tablets to break the cycle and get you back into a more normal sleep routine. Many people worry about taking sleeping tablets, and it is true that they can be addictive. However, there are times when they may be the most appropriate form of treatment, and provided you follow your doctor or pharmacist's instructions carefully, you should be able to take them for a very short period and then go back to more natural methods with no ill-effects. See Chapter 7 for more about sleeping tablets.

Even though you may not feel like socializing as such, try to stay in touch with friends and family. If you feel you'd like to talk about the person who has died, tell them this. Ask for their support while you're going through this awful period. Ask them to try not to be embarrassed or worried if you cry; so many people avoid talking about someone who has died because they fear the tears of the bereaved. There may well be tears, but that doesn't mean the sadness is greater. In fact, people looking back at the early days of their bereavement often say that talking, even if it prompted tears, helped them to come to terms with their loss more quickly. Reminiscing about happy times gone by or simply talking about how you feel about the death can help you to cope in the long run. Time is a great healer, as they say, and while it won't stop you from missing your loved one, it can help to remember that you won't always feel as bad as you do right now.

If you do not have family and friends nearby or if, despite your assurances, they find they are unable to talk with you about your loss, you may find it helpful to join a support group where you can meet and talk to others in a similar position. The knowledge that there are other people out there who understand exactly what you're going through can be immensely helpful. Cruse is a bereavement charity that offers a wide range of information, advice, support and counselling, either in groups or on a one-to-one basis. Whether you've lost a partner, sibling, friend, parent or child, and whether the death was from natural causes or as a result of suicide, accident, crime or natural disaster, Cruse will be able to offer support. See p. 108 for contact details.

The death of a loved one can be the worst thing that has ever happened to you. It will take time to recover, so don't expect too much of yourself at this difficult time. You will always feel your loss, but you *will* smile again.

5

Possible causes (physical and environmental) and solutions

If your insomnia has a physical cause – pain or illness, for example – you will need to address the particular condition as well as addressing the insomnia. This may prove easy to treat and the improvement in your sleep may be swift, or if you're unlucky it may be difficult to find a treatment that works, or that works quickly. In the first instance, though, you need to identify the cause, and this can prove difficult in some cases. This chapter will look separately at some conditions commonly associated with insomnia or poor quality sleep, and will also look at what you can do about environmental causes.

Restless legs syndrome (RLS)

The term 'restless legs syndrome' (RLS) was first used in the 1940s by Swedish neurologist Karl Ekbom to describe the sensory and motor disorder that causes a 'creepy-crawly' sensation in the legs, accompanied by a powerful urge to keep moving them. The condition, also known as Ekbom's Syndrome, is a common cause of sleep disturbance and affects around 8 per cent of adults. For some, the symptoms are mild and sleep disruption is minimal. For others, it's more severe. According to a recent study, 3 per cent of the population experience symptoms that cause 'moderate to very severe distress' at least twice a week. RLS is more common in women, and the prevalence increases with age. Symptoms range from a mild tingling or creeping sensation to pain and a powerful urge to move the legs. These symptoms usually appear when the person is at rest, and are often much worse at night, which means it can impact on partners as well.

Dr Chris Idzikowski is director of the Edinburgh Sleep Centre and often finds that people who have been referred to sleep clinics are suffering from RLS. As Dr Idzikowski explains:

RLS causes sleep disturbance and the impact of that on a person's quality of life is potentially huge. No-one functions properly if they are sleep-deprived. RLS often remains undiagnosed for some time, partly because of low awareness but also because it can be difficult to treat, especially as in many cases, it's idiopathic – meaning we don't understand what's causing it. Iron deficiency is common in those with RLS, and we often see the condition in people who give blood, so one of the first things we do is to look at checking iron levels. Pregnant women may suffer RLS, but it usually resolves after the birth. Some doctors prescribe sedatives but this is often unsuccessful because the condition tends to 'break through' the sedative. Drugs used in the treatment of Parkinson's Disease can be effective in RLS but we'd look at other options first, including 'sleep hygiene', which simply means action to promote sleep, helpful bedtime routines and so on.

Self-help

If you think you may be suffering from RLS, talk to your doctor. It's also worth contacting the Ekbom Support Group (see p. 109), which can provide information on the condition and tips on how to cope. In the meantime:

- Improve sleep by avoiding late meals and drinks containing caffeine, taking moderate, regular exercise and making your sleeping environment as quiet, dark and comfortable as possible. A warm bath and milky drink before bed may help. Avoid brain stimulation such as reading or television just before bed.
- Some medications or substances such as alcohol can make RLS worse, so take note of anything you think may be affecting you. Don't stop taking prescribed medication without talking to your doctor.
- When the sensation starts, try rubbing your legs or taking a whirlpool bath.
- A change in temperature may help – try a warm or cold bath.

Supplements

If you think your iron levels might be low, you could try taking an iron supplement. Iron supplements work best if taken with a vitamin C-rich drink such as orange juice, and this aids absorption. Research suggests that magnesium deficiency may also be a factor, and that taking a magnesium supplement may help some people. Always check with your doctor before taking dietary supplements.

Medication

A number of drugs have been used to treat RLS after clinical trials, and some, in particular dopamine agonists, have been show to be effective based on placebo-controlled randomized trials. The only drugs specifically licensed in the UK and the USA for RLS at the present time (2008) are Mirapexin (pramipexole) and Adartrel (ropinirole); both are dopamine agonists. If your RLS is particularly painful, your doctor may prescribe strong painkillers such as codeine. Other drugs that may be used include anti-epileptic drugs such as carbamazepine.

Sharon

Sharon, 42, has suffered from RLS for more than eight years. Despite numerous visits to various doctors, her condition was only diagnosed in 2005.

> It used to keep me awake almost every night, but now I've learned some self-help techniques, it's better than it was. It still drives me nuts a couple of nights a week, though. First my calves start aching, then I get a tingly, prickly feeling in my legs which makes me twitch and kick. Sometimes it can be two, three or even four hours before I get to sleep. I saw several different doctors before RLS was diagnosed. They looked for circulation problems and did blood tests, but nothing showed up, so they suggested aspirin and said that 'aches and pains' were normal. The trouble was, it was really affecting my life. Apart from the physical discomfort in my legs, I was exhausted through lack of sleep. My kicking and fidgeting also keeps my husband awake, so when I've had a bad night, we'll both have bags under our eyes in the morning. Jim's a painter and decorator and it's no fun trying to hang wallpaper after only three hours' sleep!
>
> Aspirin helped, but I didn't want to take painkillers every night, so much of the time I put up with it. Then last year a new doctor diagnosed RLS. She gave me a computer printout about the condition which

described my symptoms exactly. At last I felt someone was taking me seriously. She didn't prescribe anything, but she suggested I get in touch with the Ekbom Support Group, a self-help group for sufferers of RLS. With self-help tips from Ekbom, I'm managing to keep my RLS under control. If it starts while I'm at work, I just get up and move around. At night, it's harder to deal with. If Jim rubs my legs as soon as the sensation starts, it sometimes prevents a full attack. If that doesn't work, I get up and rub lavender massage oil into my legs, then I soak them in cold water. Sometimes I even get back into bed with freezing cold wet towels wrapped around my legs. If the pain is severe or if my legs don't calm down after a couple of hours, I'll take a painkiller. I also try to use good quality cotton bedlinen and a lightweight duvet.

Snoring

Snoring is often the subject of jokes, but you might find it difficult to see the funny side if your sleep is frequently disturbed by your own or your partner's snoring. A particularly loud snorer can reach around 90 decibels – a similar volume to that of a passing underground train. Even the average snorer registers around 60 decibels, which is about the level of normal conversation. According to the World Health Organization, the threshold for sleep disturbance is 42 decibels, and chronic night-time exposure to 50 decibels or more can cause serious health problems. Research shows that noise pollution can increase stress levels, leading to cardiovascular problems including high blood pressure and strokes.

If your snoring is caused by sleep apnoea (see p. 51), the quality of your sleep is likely to be seriously impaired. In general, however, snoring is unlikely to have a direct impact on your own sleep (unless someone wakes you up each time you snore). However, if it's keeping your partner, other family members or even your neighbours awake, it could have a significant effect on your marriage and daily life, so it is something that needs addressing.

Why do we snore?

Normally, the air we breathe through our noses passes quietly over the soft palate, down the throat and into the lungs. But when any part of this airway becomes partially or completely blocked, the soft tissues vibrate as the air passes over them, and this is what produces the sound we call snoring. While we're awake, the muscles keep the airways open, but during sleep the muscles of the mouth, nose and throat relax, causing the airway to narrow and sag as we breathe in. This narrowing of the airway, together with a blockage caused by swollen tissues, the shape of the jaw or nasal passages, or congestion caused by a cold or allergy, causes the airflow to be impeded and results in snoring.

Common causes of snoring

- Getting older – we're more likely to snore as we get older because, like all the other muscles, those in the airways become less efficient and are more likely to be flabby as we age.
- Being male – sorry, but it's true: men snore more than women, although we don't really know why. It may be partly due to the fact that women's airways are different to men's in that they are slightly less flexible. It has also been suggested that there may be hormonal factors – women are more likely to snore after they've been through the menopause, but many of those who do have found that their snoring improves after starting Hormone Replacement Therapy (HRT).
- Being overweight – excess weight is a major factor in snoring. Fatty tissue, around the neck and throat especially, will narrow the airways and lead to snoring. In fact, whether they're overweight or not, men with a collar size of 17 or more are likely to snore.
- Smoking – breathing in smoke irritates the lining of the nose and can cause congestion of the nasal passages. This means you're more likely to breathe through your mouth, and you're more likely to snore. Passive smoking – breathing in the smoke from other people's cigarettes, cigars or pipes – can also affect you.
- Alcohol – alcohol causes the muscles of the mouth and throat to relax, causing the airways to become narrowed and therefore leading to snoring. High consumption of alcohol also leads to excess weight, which is itself a factor.
- Sleeping pills – some sleeping pills act as muscle relaxants and, as we have seen, relaxed throat muscles often cause snoring.
- Sleeping position – if you sleep on your back, you're more likely to snore because your tongue may fall back into your throat,

causing an obstruction. This may be even worse if you're over-weight, because excess fat under the chin will cause the airway to narrow even further when you sleep on your back.

• Physical factors – there are a number of physical features that may make you more likely to snore: for example, the shape of your jaw, the width of your nasal passages, nasal growths or polyps, a large tongue, soft palate or uvula (the little bit of flesh that dangles at the back of your throat) or a deviated septum (where there is an abnormality in the cartilage that divides the nostrils). All of these can obstruct your breathing and lead to snoring. A simple examination may reveal the cause, and in some cases it may be possible to resolve this with a routine surgical procedure.

What can you do about it?

There are a number of simple changes you can make that may improve the situation; for example, if you're overweight, start adjusting your diet so that you eat more fresh fruit and vegetables and fewer sugary and fatty foods. This, together with gradually increasing your daily exercise, should help you lose weight without too much trouble. You already know the health risks of smoking, and snoring is just one more problem to add to the list, so if you're having trouble giving up, talk to your doctor about getting some help. As noted earlier, many surgeries in the UK now have 'quit clinics' and can offer free advice and practical support to help you stop. Try cutting down the amount of alcohol you drink; even a moderate intake can increase the likelihood of snoring. If your snoring is linked to alcohol, avoid drinking for the last couple of hours before bed. If you find you tend to sleep on your back, try sleeping on your side instead. If you move onto your back while asleep, ask your partner to give you a (gentle) dig in the ribs when you start to snore in the hope that you automatically shift position without waking up. You could also try stitching a tennis ball (some people suggest a pine cone!) to the back of your pyjama top to discourage you from rolling onto your back.

If your snoring is caused by nasal congestion, you need to find out what's causing it. Obviously you'll know if you have a cold and the situation will probably resolve when you're better, but if the congestion persists it may be that you've developed an allergy. Common causes are:

- Dust – a cocktail of materials, many of which are potentially allergenic: fibres from various types of fabric, particles from plants and insects, mould spores, fur, animal 'dander' – flakes of skin covered in dried sweat and saliva – and, probably the most common household allergen, the dust mite.
- Dust mites – microscopic creatures that feed on human and animal dander. Just half a teaspoonful of dust can contain anything from 500 to several thousand mites, all producing droppings which cause the allergic reaction. Dust mites love warm, dark and humid conditions and thrive in carpets and soft furnishings. They're present in every house, especially warm, poorly ventilated houses.
- Pets – although dog and cat hair may cause a reaction, research shows that the main allergen is in fact proteins in the animal's sweat, saliva and urine.

If you think your congestion may be due to an allergy, try these tips:

- Keep your home well ventilated and turn the central heating down whenever possible, especially in bedrooms.
- Keep dust at bay by replacing carpets with wood floors or non-fibre coverings where possible. Consider swapping heavy curtains for wipe-clean blinds.
- Carpets and soft furnishings are havens for dust mites, so vacuum regularly and thoroughly.
- Dust surfaces and hard floors with a damp cloth so dust doesn't fly around.
- Wash all bedding weekly in hot (60°C, 140°F) water.
- Turn and vacuum your mattress regularly.
- Keep pets out of bedrooms and off the furniture.
- Consider buying allergy-reducing products. According to Allergy UK (contact details on p. 107), the three products that tend to be the most useful in reducing household allergens are: mattress covers and dust-mite-proof pillowcases; a good, powerful vacuum cleaner; and an air-purifier filter.

Anti-snoring products

There are a number of products on the market that claim varying degrees of success in stopping or reducing snoring. These include nasal sprays, strips and dilators, oral appliances designed to hold the jaw and tongue forward, shields to prevent mouth-breathing and, for those with sleep apnoea, Continuous Positive Airway Pressure (CPAP) machines (see p. 53). The suitability of these products will depend on what type of snorer you are – in other words, whether your snoring is due to a larger-than-average tongue or palate, narrowed nasal passages, mouth-breathing or the shape of your jaw, or whether you are suffering from sleep apnoea. The British Snoring and Sleep Apnoea Association (BSSAA) has a large selection of these products and offers advice, via their website or over the telephone, on how to assess what type of snorer you are and how to choose the most appropriate product. See p. 108 for their contact details.

Sleep apnoea

Snoring is annoying, but it doesn't usually have serious implications for the physical health of the snorer. Sleep apnoea, however, can have a serious impact on health and can even be life-threatening. It is a cause of snoring, but relatively few snorers suffer from sleep apnoea, and some people with sleep apnoea hardly snore at all. *Apnoea* is a Greek word meaning 'without breath', and describes the periods where the sleeper literally stops breathing for ten seconds or more. When this happens, oxygen levels in the blood fall sharply and the brain goes into emergency mode, releasing a surge of adrenaline into the system to wake you up, often with a loud snore, snort or choking noise, so that you breathe again. This is classed as 'clinically significant' when it happens more than ten times an hour. Even though you won't be aware of waking up dozens, possibly hundreds, of times a night, you will clearly feel the effects of such profoundly disturbed sleep, and one of the main symptoms of the condition is daytime sleepiness. Other symptoms include: feeling unrefreshed after what appears to have been a full night's sleep, lack of concentration, irritability, problems with memory, morning headaches and dry mouth. Sleep apnoea is often only picked up after the person's partner notices that he or she stops breathing during the night.

Sleepiness and poor concentration caused by sleep apnoea can lead to reduced reaction times, making accidents more likely. The condition is thought to be a factor in a significant number of accidents at work, in the home and on the roads – someone with the condition is roughly seven times more likely to have a road accident. This means that not only is the person with sleep apnoea at risk, but so are members of the wider public who may be involved in an accident that occurs as a result of the condition. Other risks associated with sleep apnoea include hypertension (high blood pressure), heart problems and strokes. This is thought to be due to the repeated falls in blood oxygen levels. It is therefore extremely important to see your doctor if you think there's any chance you might have this condition.

If you are diagnosed with sleep apnoea, you must inform the Driver and Vehicle Licensing Agency (DVLA). If you don't, you could be fined up to £1,000 and your insurance will be invalidated. If there is excessive daytime sleepiness, you will not be allowed to drive again until you can show (usually though a doctor's report) that your symptoms are properly under control.

Types of sleep apnoea

The most common type of sleep apnoea is Obstructive Sleep Apnoea (OSA). As we have seen, snoring is often the result of narrowed airways causing inhaled air to make a noise as it hits the soft, relaxed tissues at the back of the throat. In OSA, the airway collapses in on itself, becoming completely blocked. When this happens, breathing stops and then restarts more than ten seconds later. The sleeper may appear to choke or gasp for air, which can be quite alarming for a partner witnessing the episode. Far less common is Central Sleep Apnoea (CSA). This is where the brain fails to send the 'breathe now' signal to your body while you're sleeping. A third type, Mixed Sleep Apnoea (MSA), is a combination of OSA and CSA.

What can be done?

If you suspect you may have sleep apnoea, following the advice in the previous section on snoring may help – sleeping on your side, losing weight, or lifestyle changes such as giving up smoking and cutting down on alcohol, especially in the evenings, for example (see p. 49). The next thing to do is to see your doctor and get a diagnosis. This may take some time, because if your doctor suspects sleep apnoea he or she will probably refer you to a sleep clinic. This allows the specialist to observe you and carry out a number of tests while you sleep (more about sleep clinics in Chapter 7). The treatment you're offered will depend on the severity of your sleep apnoea. This is measured in various ways, but the doctors will be particularly interested in the number of apnoeas you suffer per hour. As a rough guide, if it's between five and 20 per hour, you have mild sleep apnoea; if it's between 20 and 35, you have moderate sleep apnoea, and if it's more than 35 per hour, your sleep apnoea is classed as severe. Doctors will also take into account the levels of your daytime sleepiness. Do you just doze off watching television, for example, or do you fall asleep in the middle of a meal, while talking to someone or even while driving?

If you're suffering from severe sleep apnoea, doctors may recommend a Continuous Positive Airway Pressure (CPAP) machine. This is an air pump with a mask attached that you wear over your nose or mouth and nose while you sleep. The pump blows slightly pressurized air into your throat, the pressure acting as an air splint to keep your airway open. A number of studies have concluded that CPAP machines are the most effective treatment for severe sleep apnoea, with people reporting more refreshing sleep and significantly less daytime sleepiness. So far, there has not been enough research to indicate whether the use of a CPAP machine can reduce the risk of hypertension and heart disease associated with sleep apnoea. On the downside, some people find the mask uncomfortable and difficult to use. It also causes side effects in some people, including dry mouth, nose and throat, sneezing or a blocked or runny nose, sore eyes and chest discomfort. However, most people find that even if they do experience side effects, these are easier to cope with than the effects of the sleep apnoea. Often, people who struggle with the CPAP machine at first find that persevering with the device really pays off, and after a couple of weeks they wonder how they survived without it!

Deborah

As a nurse working on a respiratory ward, Deborah, 25, already knew a little about sleep apnoea and she'd helped some of her patients get used to using a CPAP machine, so she knew what to expect when she was herself diagnosed with the condition. Deborah says:

> My mum said I snored even as a child, but it was only when my husband noticed that I would often stop breathing while I was asleep that I realized I might have sleep apnoea. I'd been feeling tired during the day for a long time. I'd wake in the morning feeling as though I'd hardly slept, then I'd crawl through the day, just wanting to lie down and sleep. When I got home from work, I'd sit on the sofa and fall asleep immediately. It got to the point where I couldn't watch television or even read a book without nodding off. Eventually, I was referred to a consultant who diagnosed sleep apnoea and recommended a CPAP machine. I was probably less apprehensive than some people because I knew all about CPAP machines as some of my patients used them. Having said that, it did take a few days to get used to. I found it a bit uncomfortable at first because I have eczema and the mask aggravated my skin, but then they gave me a gel mask, which is much more comfortable. Using the machine made a difference to how I felt very quickly. Within a couple of weeks, I had more energy, felt much less tired and found it easier to get up – I felt as though I'd actually slept!
>
> I've been using the machine for two years now and I wouldn't be without it. I have a check-up every six months and my condition has definitely improved, partly, I think, because I've lost a lot of weight, but mainly due to the CPAP machine. The one I have is quite an old model and measures about 15 cm by 15 cm, so it takes up a bit of room on the bedside table, but the ones they're bringing out now are much smaller and less obtrusive. I haven't really had side effects apart from an occasional headache, which may or may not be a side effect of using the machine, but even if it is I feel so much better in general that I'm happy to put up with the odd headache!

Other treatments

Wearing a mouthpiece that pushes your jaw slightly forward may help to keep your airway open. The device fits around your teeth and is a bit like the gumshields used by some sportspeople. There is not a lot of research on mouthpieces so far, but doctors generally agree that they can help. Side effects include dry mouth, gum irritation and dribbling, although these usually improve after the first week or two.

Surgery

Depending on what doctors think is causing your sleep apnoea, surgery may be an option, especially if you find using a CPAP machine too uncomfortable or intrusive. Surgery for sleep apnoea focuses on correcting the obstruction of the upper airway. Obstruction of the upper airway can occur at several levels including the palate, the base of the tongue or both. There may also be nasal obstruction, but while this can contribute to the tendency for the airway to collapse, it is rarely the sole cause of sleep apnoea. Surgery is aimed at correcting whichever obstruction is present, thus enlarging the airway. This often involves trimming and tightening throat tissues while you are under a general anaesthetic. However, this procedure has only a 20–50 per cent success rate, and although not complicated or dangerous, it is quite painful during recovery. Surgery for sleep apnoea is usually regarded as a last resort.

Pregnancy

It has been suggested that insomnia during pregnancy is nature's way of preparing women for motherhood! If you're expecting a baby, you're likely to feel more tired than usual, especially in the early months, and yet this is when you're most likely to suffer disturbed sleep. This may be due to frequent urination because of the pressure on the bladder caused by the expanding uterus. The pressure increases and you need the loo more often, which can lead to wakefulness. Drink plenty during the day, but avoid too much liquid just before bed, and empty your bladder last thing before you put the light out. Nausea can also keep you awake, or wake you during the night. It's called 'morning sickness' but it can affect you at any time of day or night. Try eating small, regular snacks rather than big meals, and sip ginger tea whenever you're affected. Hormonal changes and breast tenderness can also keep you awake at night, although these tend to settle down after the first few weeks. The good news is that the second trimester (three to six months) is often a period of good quality sleep and increased daytime energy. Unfortunately, this is soon eclipsed by the problems of the third trimester, when your sheer bulk can make sleeping, or even getting comfortable, difficult. There may also be more pressure on your bladder in this trimester, or you may suffer from heartburn, restless legs (see p. 44) or snoring (see p. 47). Talk to your midwife about any problems and follow the general advice for a healthy pregnancy: eat the best diet you can, take moderate exercise and, if you're not getting a good night's sleep, take short naps during the day.

Wakeful children

New mums are probably among the most sleep-deprived members of society. They may sleep for only an hour or two at a time, totting up a night's total of just four or five hours (on a good night!). Those of us who went through all this years ago look back now and wonder how we did it, but we survived. Even when night feeds are no longer an issue, your baby may not sleep for long stretches of time, or not at the same time as you want to sleep. Toddlers tend to sleep better than babies, and school-age children better still. But there are many things that can affect your child's – and therefore your own – ability to sleep through the night. These may include daytime naps, coughs and colds, nightmares, aches and pains, bed-wetting or fears and anxieties. A regular bedtime routine usually helps a child to settle, and there are a number of steps you can take to help a child who wakes during the night; however, you may find that even when your child sleeps through, you're so used to waking up or being awake that you find it difficult to get back into your usual, pre-parenthood pattern of sleep. So it's a double problem: first, you have to help your child have a good night's sleep, then you have to help yourself. Wakeful children are such a common cause of sleep disturbance that the whole of Chapter 9 is devoted to the subject, and you will find some tips there to help you cope with some of the more common issues affecting children's sleep. If you find yourself suffering from insomnia even once the children are sleeping well, it may be that you have become 'conditioned' to expect wakefulness. If this is the case, some simple self-help steps may be enough to resolve the situation. See Chapter 6 for advice on how to get the best night's sleep you possibly can.

Menopause

It is quite common for women to find that their sleep difficulties begin or worsen in the few years leading up to the menopause. This may be due to the significant changes in hormone levels, it may be to do with hot flushes and night sweats or it may be a combination of these. It is also around this time that many women experience major life changes such as bereavement, divorce or children leaving home, all of which can cause anxiety, depression and sleeplessness. It may be that you need help in coping with these changes (see Chapter 4 for tips on coping with insomnia related to stress, depression and anxiety) or it may be more appropriate to treat the possible physical causes. For many women, Hormone Replacement Therapy (HRT) brings about a dramatic improvement in their insomnia and in other symptoms, such as hot flushes and night sweats, that may contribute to it. As you will be aware, there are a number of pros and cons involved in taking HRT, so you need to discuss the potential benefits and risks with your doctor before deciding whether you'd like to try it. If you decide that HRT is not for you, there are other options. Herbal remedies such as red clover and black cohosh work well for some women, and a diet rich in phytoestrogens can also be beneficial. Phytoestrogens are plant oestrogens which have a similar, though much weaker, effect to human oestrogen. Foods containing phytoestrogens include soya beans and tofu (soya bean-curd), flaxseed, linseed, pulses (especially lentils and chickpeas), celery, bean sprouts, rhubarb, grains and citrus fruits.

If you are particularly troubled by hot flushes and night sweats, these tips may help:

- Avoid alcohol or hot drinks, especially just before going to bed.
- Wear loose cotton nightwear (or none at all).

- Use good quality cotton bedlinen. Sheets and blankets may be better than a duvet, as you can easily peel off a layer or two when you need to.
- Keep a spray bottle of water (like a perfume spray) by your bed. When you feel yourself heating up, spray a fine mist onto your face, neck and the insides of your wrists.
- Sleep with the window open if possible.
- Make some sage tea by steeping a teaspoonful of chopped sage leaves in boiling water. Allow the tea to cool and sip it through the night.

Also, see Chapter 6 for general tips on how to get a good night's sleep.

Bedroom not conducive to sleep

As mentioned previously, sleep experts often say that the bedroom, especially the bed, should be used for only two things, sleep and sex – although a bedtime read is probably allowed, as long as the book isn't too exciting! What they're really getting at is the tendency to use the bedroom as a second living room, with television sets, DVD players and music systems now commonplace in many a bedroom. When you can't sleep, the temptation to watch a film or catch up on the soaps is quite strong, but these stimulating distractions will actually make sleep even more elusive. If you use a corner of your bedroom as a home office, you're unlikely to be able to switch off properly from work while you're in bed. If you have a computer in your bedroom, not only will you be tempted to surf the net when you can't sleep, but the very presence of a machine you use for work or for household administration can remind you, even if only at a subconscious level, of stressful activity.

The room in which you sleep should be as relaxing as possible. You can create an environment conducive to sleep by clearing out the media gadgets, painting the walls in a calming colour, and making sure the room is the right temperature and as dark and quiet as possible. See p. 64 for more details on how to create the optimum sleep environment.

Long-term illness

Insomnia can also be due to an underlying illness such as an over-active thyroid. Any condition that causes pain, such as arthritis or backache, is likely to affect your ability to sleep, as is anything that causes breathing problems, such as asthma or heart failure. Gastrointestinal disorders such as heartburn or indigestion can make sleep difficult. It may also be possible that your insomnia is a side effect of medication you take for another condition – some painkillers contain caffeine, for example. Talk to your doctor or pharmacist about this; there may be another suitable medicine you can take.

Noisy environment

Noise is one of the most common environmental causes of sleep disturbance. Earplugs may help. They're quite comfortable once you get used to them, and although they reduce the amount of noise they don't block it out completely, so you don't need to worry that you wouldn't hear a crying child. If you live on a busy main road, it might be worth changing rooms so that the room you sleep in is furthest away from the source of noise. If you have noisy neighbours, try having a diplomatic chat with them. It's best not to go round when the noise is actually happening, because if you're feeling angry or stressed it'll be difficult to make a relaxed, polite request. It may be that your neighbours don't realize that their noise is disturbing you, in which case a friendly chat might solve the problem. However, if you're unlucky enough to have neighbours who are particularly anti-social, talking to them could make matters worse. Or it may be that they simply won't listen. Noise nuisance from neighbours, whether the premises are domestic or commercial, is unacceptable and if it continues to be a serious problem they can be prosecuted. Keep a record of the dates, duration and levels of noise (e.g. 'music so loud we could hear the lyrics even above the sound of our television') and talk to your local Environmental Health department. They will advise you on what to do next.

If you can't do anything about the noise, you could try changing your attitude towards it. It can sometimes be how you *feel* about the noise that keeps you awake – it's very hard to sleep when you're feeling anywhere between mildly irritated and downright furious. People can sometimes train themselves to sleep through quite high levels of noise. Use relaxation exercises (see p. 71) to calm yourself and help yourself relax. It may also help to listen to some soothing music while you drop off, in order to mask other noise.

Jet lag

Travelling by plane frequently, whether it's for work or leisure, can upset your circadian rhythms or 'body clock'. When you cross into another time zone this biological mechanism takes a while to catch up, and this can alter your normal sleep patterns. The effect is similar to that experienced by shift workers, especially those who work both night and day shifts. Some people cope better with these changes than others, but if you find that jet lag frequently disrupts your sleep, you can sometimes minimize the effects. There is some evidence to suggest that taking melatonin, the sleep hormone, is useful in treating jet lag. However, there is also research that indicates the contrary. Experts are currently divided on whether melatonin is an appropriate treatment, and many agree that we don't yet know enough about the potential side effects or the long-term effects on health. There are other steps you can take to help ease the symptoms:

- Before you go, try to reset your body clock by following a plan of carefully timed exposure to light and dark – exposure to light at the wrong time can actually make jet lag worse. Your personal plan will depend on a number of factors including your destination, the time of day or night you will be travelling, how many time zones you'll be crossing and whether you are normally a 'lark' or an 'owl'. To work out what's best for you, visit one of the websites that offer free body-clock calculators, for example <www.bodyclock.com>. If you don't have the internet at home, remember you can always access it at an internet café or, usually free, at a public library.
- If you're travelling at night, try to get some sleep on the plane. Take earplugs, an eye mask and a comfortable head and neck

support pillow. Fly business or first class if you can afford it – improved comfort means you're more likely to be able to sleep.

- Avoid alcohol and caffeinated drinks, eat light meals and drink plenty of water. Stretch frequently or get up and walk around if you can.
- When you arrive, try to fit in straight away with your destination's sleep–wake pattern. So if you arrive in the morning, expose yourself to daylight and try to stay awake even if you're tired; take a 15-minute nap if you need to. If you arrive in the evening, go to bed at an hour that's not too much later than your normal bedtime. You'll probably still feel groggy for a while, but you'll readjust more quickly.

6

Help yourself to get a good night's sleep

Keeping a sleep diary

Keeping a diary of your sleep–wake pattern and the various things that affect it can be valuable in assessing the extent and possible causes or factors involved in your sleep patterns. Often, we tend not to notice subtle changes in our daily habits and routines, but these changes can affect our sleep and so recording these things in a diary will help to show up any adverse effects.

The most effective way to keep a sleep diary is to do so over a period of at least two weeks when you don't need to set your alarm clock. Try to record any information that might be relevant. You'll need two separate records, one to be completed in the morning when you wake, and one to be completed before bed in the evening.

How to complete the diary

Use two large sheets of paper and write the days of the week along the top of each page, and then on the left of the first sheet list each hour from your usual waking time until your usual bedtime, e.g. 7 a.m.–11 p.m. Then, on the second sheet, list the hours of the night, say midnight to 6 a.m. Use a ruler to draw lines down and across to form a grid. Complete the diary with as much relevant information as you can fit in, including the time you actually get into bed as well as the time (roughly) you fall asleep. For the times when you're actually asleep in bed, shade the relevant boxes with a pencil; use a different colour to shade the boxes where you have only slept for part of the hour (include naps). You could write in here 'dozed in chair for ten mins' or whatever. Other information can be recorded in detail, e.g. '1 p.m. – lunch: cheese on toast, apple, cup of tea, chocolate biscuit', or with an abbreviation, for example

'C' for a cup of coffee or 'A' for an alcoholic drink. When you wake in the night, take note of the time and then, in the morning, you can record it in your diary, together with the reason for waking, e.g. '3 a.m. N' (noise) or 'T' (toilet). Make sure you record your activities as well, especially the things you do in the evening: for example, going for a walk, going out with friends, reading, watching television, having a bath. If you take any medication to help you sleep, whether it's prescribed or 'over-the-counter', record this as well. If you feel particularly sleepy during the day, note this and when or if it improved, for example after a walk or a nap.

Keep the diary for at least two weeks, after which you can use the information you've gathered to help tackle your sleep issues. Some of the things that might be helpful are: diet – are there any particular foods or drinks that keep you awake, give you indigestion or cause you to wake frequently to empty your bladder? Does going to the gym or for a walk in the evening help you go to sleep earlier or make it more difficult to settle? Maybe you should take your exercise earlier in the evening. Look at the times you go to bed and get up, and compare them with the times you fall asleep and the times you wake. If you have trouble getting to sleep, maybe you should go to bed slightly later. As a rule, you shouldn't spend much longer than 20 minutes in bed awake, so if you're putting the light out at 11 p.m. but your diary shows you are frequently awake until midnight, a later bedtime might be appropriate. The same applies if you wake earlier than you plan to get up. Forcing yourself to stay in bed and trying to get back to sleep can make you feel worse in the long run than simply getting up and getting on with the day a little earlier. Obviously, this depends on the time you wake – if you don't go to sleep until after midnight and you wake at four, it's clearly too early to start the day. As a general rule, you should spend at least five hours in bed. If that's all you can manage but you still feel tired during the day, try to extend your sleep duration very gradually, going to bed 10 minutes earlier and getting up 10 minutes later for the first week, then 20 minutes for the second week and so on. Hopefully, you'll be able to train your body to drop off sooner and stay asleep for longer. If the diary shows that you tend to wake during the night and don't go back to sleep for an hour, you could try getting up after 20 minutes and going into another room. Don't do anything too stimulating, just relax away from the bedroom and return as soon as you start to feel sleepy.

Your sleep diary should help you to see what's causing or contributing to your sleep difficulties; it can also be a useful tool for your doctor or specialist, should you need further help.

To nap or not to nap?

You've probably read a number of articles in newspapers and magazines advising you against taking a daytime nap if you're having trouble sleeping. It's certainly true that going to bed for two hours in the afternoon to 'make up' for having lost a couple of hours' sleep at night can make matters worse. If you sleep for too long in the day, you won't be sleepy at your normal bedtime, so you'll stay awake later than usual, feel awful in the morning because you've had a short night and so be tempted to take another nap. In other words, you've set up a vicious circle. However, there is significant evidence to suggest that a *short* nap during the day may be beneficial, both in terms of creativity and productivity and in terms of overall health. Professor Jim Horne of the Sleep Research Centre at Loughborough University recommends a nap of around 15 minutes. 'Most credible sleep experts agree,' says Professor Horne. 'A short nap in the daytime when you feel sleepy can be very effective.'

The perfect sleep environment

Many people find that they sleep better when they're away from home. If you're on holiday, it probably has a lot to do with the fact that you're away from the stresses and strains of your job and the usual daily domestic responsibilities. However, it can also have something to do with your sleep environment. If you've ever stayed in a really good hotel, the chances are you had a pretty good night's sleep. Just think about that big comfy bed, freshly laundered sheets, soft pillows, squashy duvet. The room is clean and tidy – no piles of ironing or papers, no games consul or computer winking at you from the corner. The television and other gadgets are hidden away in a cupboard, no-one's going to telephone or email and there's nothing to remind you of the stresses of the rest of the day. Adjacent to your room is a pristine bathroom with a basket of luxury toiletries and a heated rail draped with soft, fluffy towels, so before bed you treat yourself to a long fragrant soak. Having wrapped yourself in warm towels, you draw the heavy curtains blocking out any light from outside, then you slip between the cool, fresh sheets and drift off happily to the Land of Nod.

Ah, sounds good, doesn't it? Sadly, few of us can afford to stay in top hotels very often, if ever. But you can improve your sleep environment so that it's at least a little nearer to this sleep-friendly ideal. First, remove television and computer equipment. As previously mentioned, the bedroom should be for sleep and sex only. Anything lying around to do with work or anything remotely stressful – piles of household bills, for example – should be banished to another room. Your bedroom should be as dark as you can make it, so fit heavy curtains or blackout blinds. It should also be the correct temperature. It can be tempting to whack up the central heating on a cold night, but this really isn't conducive to good sleep. In fact, most experts suggest that somewhere between 16 and 18 degrees Celsius (60 and 65 degrees Fahrenheit) is the ideal.

The right bed

We spend roughly a third of our lives in bed, so it really is worth getting it right. An uncomfortable or worn-out bed can contribute to sleep difficulties, so you should think about whether you need to buy a new one. If your bed is more than ten years old, you should definitely replace it. Even if it's not that old, can you feel the springs? Does the bed creak when you move around? Do you and your partner tend to roll together (without meaning to)? If so, you should consider buying a new one.

Buy the best bed you can afford and allow yourself plenty of time to choose it. Professor Chris Idzikowski of the Sleep Assessment and Advisory Service recommends you check with the sales assistant that you will be able to test the bed for up to 30 minutes – if the shop objects, walk away. The bed should not be too soft but, contrary to popular belief, it shouldn't be too firm either. The way to test this is to lie on your back and slide your hand into the hollow near the base of your spine. If your hand slides in easily, the bed may be too firm;

if you can't slide your hand in, it's too soft. Another thing you need to consider is the size of your bed. We toss and turn up to 70 times a night, and if you share your bed with a partner you can hardly avoid disturbing each other, especially if your bed is on the small side. Consider buying a king-size bed, which is usually around 152 cm (60 inches) wide and 198 cm (78 inches) long, though this can vary from manufacturer to manufacturer. If your sleep is frequently disturbed because of your partner tossing and turning, you may want to consider buying a 'zip and link' bed – essentially two single beds that can be zipped together, so when one partner turns over, the other will barely be aware of it. This type of bed is also a good solution if you and your partner are very different in terms of weight.

Making up the bed

Good quality cotton bedlinen is usually more comfortable to sleep on and will allow your skin to breathe. If you tend to get too hot during the night, make your bed up in layers so that you can throw them off and pull them back on when necessary. If you use a duvet, make sure you're using one that'll provide the best comfort possible. Duvets filled with natural fibres are best as they absorb moisture – we sweat up to half a pint of fluid a night. You also need to consider how warm you want the duvet to be, and how heavy. In general, the higher the tog rating, the warmer the duvet. As a rough guide:

- Lightweight summer duvet 4.5 tog;
- Spring and autumn medium-weight duvet 9.0–10.5 tog;
- Winter heavyweight duvet 12.0–13.5 tog.

One solution is to buy two duvets, one lightweight and one medium-weight, and then to use them both together in the winter. You can buy duvets made for this purpose that can be joined together with press-studs. If you want a warm duvet but prefer a lighter weight, a down filling might be the best option. Goose down is lighter than duck, but more expensive. If you like a heavier duvet to snuggle under, consider a down and feather mix or a good quality synthetic.

The right pillow is also important because it can affect the alignment of your body. Your pillow should provide support for your neck as well as your head and maintain a straight line between your neck and spine. If your pillow doesn't do this, or if it's more than a couple of years old, you should buy a new one. If you sleep on your side, you'll need a plump, firm pillow to give you the best neck and shoulder support. If you sleep on your back, a medium firm pillow will suit you better, and if you tend to sleep on your front, go for a softer pillow as this will cushion your head and neck at a comfortable angle.

Diet – sleep saboteurs

You're less likely to have trouble sleeping if you have a healthy diet and avoid large meals for two or three hours before bedtime. Different foods affect people in different ways, so the best way to find out exactly how your diet affects your sleep is to include a record of everything you eat and drink in your sleep diary (see p. 62). This will help you to identify the foods that might be stopping you from sleeping properly.

Caffeine

One of the most common sleep disrupters, caffeine is present not just in coffee but in tea, drinking chocolate, cocoa and some fizzy drinks, especially some 'energy' drinks. It's also present in some painkillers, over-the-counter stimulants and herbal preparations, so you really do need to start checking the labels of everything you consume. Caffeine is a powerful stimulant that enters the bloodstream very quickly and stays in the body for between three and seven hours. Some people can take quite large amounts of caffeine and still sleep well; others find that just one cup of coffee in the morning affects their sleep that night. Experts suggest this may be because some people are particularly sensitive to caffeine and their bodies seem to metabolize the caffeine more slowly.

The worst offenders are coffee, tea and some cola or energy drinks. Percolated coffee usually contains more caffeine than instant powders and granules; tea brewed with leaves has more caffeine than that made with a tea bag; and plain chocolate contains more caffeine than milk chocolate.

Alcohol

One of the most common sleep myths is that an alcoholic 'nightcap' will help you to get a good night's sleep. In fact, the reverse is true. While a few drinks may help you to nod off, the immediate effects will wear off after three or four hours and you're likely to experienced disrupted, fitful sleep for the rest of the night. Alcohol is a diuretic, so you're more likely to wake up several times to use the loo when you've been drinking. Alcohol also impairs breathing, so you're more likely to snore. The effects of alcohol will be enhanced if you're sleep-deprived, so beware of drinking too much in desperation when you're really tired. This is not to say you have to stop drinking completely – a small amount of alcohol is associated with a number of health benefits – but do try to stay within safe drinking limits (current government guidelines recommend no more than 3–4 units a day for men and 2–3 for women). Use your sleep diary to increase your awareness of the effect alcohol has on your sleep.

One unit of alcohol is roughly equivalent to:

- half a pint of normal-strength beer or lager;
- a small glass (125 ml) of wine;
- a pub measure (25 ml) of spirits;
- half a glass (50 ml) of fortified wine such as port or sherry.

Many bottles now bear labels that tell you how many units of alcohol that bottle contains.

Sugar

Sugar can disrupt sleep because of its effect on blood-sugar levels. If too much sugar is released into the bloodstream, the effect is an instant 'high', followed by a sharp drop. This can make you feel hungry again quite quickly, and it also causes a rise in the levels of adrenaline, the hormone associated with wakefulness. Fluctuating blood-sugar levels can leave you feeling exhausted but unable to sleep, so you need to try and keep the levels fairly steady. The best way to achieve this is to eat little and often during the day, avoiding foods that are high in fat and sugar, and eating more foods containing 'complex' carbohydrates, for example vegetables, wholemeal breads and cereals, beans, lentils, chickpeas, barley, oats, brown rice and root vegetables. These foods release energy into the bloodstream more slowly, helping you to go for longer periods without becoming hungry. A small, complex-carb snack a couple of hours before bed will help sustain you through the night. Try a couple of oatcakes or a wholemeal sandwich; a milky drink may help, too, but avoid anything chocolate-based that may contain caffeine.

Diet – sleep enhancers

Some foods and drinks do seem to help. Magnesium- and calcium-rich foods help to induce calmness. Milk is an excellent calcium source, while nuts, seeds, pulses and green vegetables are good for magnesium. Camomile tea is widely thought to have relaxing, sleep-promoting qualities. Other teas that may help include wild lettuce, passionflower and lemon balm. Foods rich in tryptophan can be a good evening meal choice; tryptophan is converted into serotonin, which in turn converts into melatonin, the sleepiness hormone. Turkey, bananas, milk, nuts and dried apricots all contain high levels of tryptophan, and starchy carbohydrates such as whole-grain cereals also increase production of serotonin. Lettuce contains lactucarium, which is a natural sedative. Eat the leaves raw, make lettuce soup or drink as an infusion in the evenings.

Exercise

We all know that exercise is important for general health. Not only does it reduce the risk of heart disease and other diseases but it will help keep your joints, bones and muscles strong and healthy. Exercise can also improve mood and reduce your risk of depression – another condition that can affect your ability to sleep. Lack of sleep has been shown to increase the risk of obesity and, of course, regular exercise can help to reduce that risk.

The trouble is, if you're having difficulty sleeping you may well feel too tired to exercise, especially after a particularly bad night. However, it really is worth making the initial effort, because you'll feel an almost immediate boost in energy that will help you get through the day and help you to sleep better at night. Research suggests that regular, moderate exercise has a beneficial effect on sleep. A recent study in a group of people over 65 found that 30–40 minutes of brisk walking four times a week resulted in a significant improvement. Participants reported falling asleep more quickly and staying asleep for longer periods.

Make sure you find something you enjoy doing. A combination of aerobic exercise, which will get the heart and lungs working, and stretching, which in turn will help you relax, is ideal. Many people find that joining a gym not only helps them to get fit but is also an opportunity to meet new people, thus adding an extra dimension to their social lives. Others prefer individual activities such as walking, running or cycling. Whatever you choose and however quickly you feel the benefits, it is important to fit exercise into your life on a regular basis. Half an hour's aerobic exercise at least three or four times a week should make a difference both to your overall health and to your ability to sleep. Exercise in the fresh air is particularly beneficial, and a brisk daily walk will improve your fitness and calm the mind. Find a time that you can fit in on a regular basis. If the only time you can exercise is in the evening, make it fairly early – the initial effect of exercise is an energy boost, so just before bed is not ideal!

Lifestyle and sleep

As we've seen, taking regular exercise and making changes to your diet can improve your sleep. But are there any other changes you could make to your lifestyle that would help you to sleep better? Do you need to look at your social life, for example? Dancing till dawn and generally being a party animal is all well and good if you can sleep half the day to make up for it. But if you have to get back into the swing of a 9–5 (or 12–8, or whatever) existence, frequent late nights will throw your body clock out of kilter and make it more difficult for you to resume a normal sleep pattern. If you are suffering from sleep disruption or excessive daytime tiredness, try to stick to a more regular routine. The odd late night won't do you any harm, and a short nap (15–20 minutes) the following day will help you to stay on top of things, but if you let the late nights build up the situation could be more difficult to sort out.

The internet can be a very disruptive influence on sleep. Because of its 24/7 nature, you can do your banking, pay bills, gamble, shop or chat to friends and strangers at any time. There are forums and 'chat rooms' on any topic you can think of, and staying up 'talking' can become addictive. Do keep a check on your internet use, as this sort of activity can make it difficult to fall asleep when you finally log off.

For many people, it is work rather than play that is the biggest sleep disrupter. Bringing your work home with you may sometimes be unavoidable, but if you allow work worries to occupy your mind right up until bedtime, you'll find it difficult to switch off when you need to. It may be that you simply have too much to do, and if you're tired you'll find it even harder. Struggling through on short nights of broken sleep can have serious detrimental effects on your memory, decision-making and general efficiency, so you won't be able to cope with the same workload as someone who is well rested. If stopping work two hours earlier each evening helps you to relax before bed and therefore to sleep better, it's quite likely that you'll achieve more in an eight-hour day than you previously achieved in ten hours. Learning how to relax properly is also important, as is getting into good bedtime habits, sometimes called 'sleep hygiene'. See the quick reference guide on p. 77 for sleep hygiene tips. To help you unwind, try this simple relaxation exercise.

Lie flat on your back with your legs straight and uncrossed, and your arms loosely at your sides. With your eyes closed and starting with your feet, tense each group of muscles (see box) and, after a count of ten, relax them and allow them to go limp. Give yourself a few moments between each muscle group and continue until you reach your head. Your breathing should be even and natural, not too shallow. With a bit of luck, you'll nod off before you even get that far.

Major muscle groups

Hips and legs – feet, calves, thighs, buttocks.
Torso – lower back, abdomen, stomach, chest.
Arms – hands, forearms, upper arms (biceps).
Head and shoulders – shoulders, neck, throat, head.
Face – jaw, tongue, lips, nose, cheeks, eyes, brow.

Sex and sleep

Kissing, cuddling or giving one another a massage after a long day can help relieve stress, making you feel more relaxed and sleepy. This kind of physical intimacy helps you to feel loved and secure, which makes it easier to relax. And if the intimacy leads to sex, so much the better, because this triggers the release of endorphins which cause the body and mind to relax deeply. Sex also improves circulation, which helps to remove waste products that could cause fatigue. It can also help you live longer – a ten-year study of 1,000 middle-aged men by Queen's University in Belfast found that men of similar age and health who had frequent orgasms had half of the death rate of those who didn't. Researchers believe this is due to reduction in stress associated with frequent sexual activity.

Deep breathing and meditation

It is very difficult to relax effectively if you don't get your breathing right. Breathing is usually an unconscious action, but because we never think about it, many of us breathe incorrectly. Take a deep breath now – has your chest risen? What about your stomach and abdomen? If only your chest rises when you breathe in, this indicates shallow breathing. Deeper breathing is slower than shallow breathing and will help to slow your heart rate and calm your mind. Here's how to do it.

Lie on your back with one hand on your chest, the other on your abdomen. Begin to breathe in slowly through your nose, allowing your lungs to expand. Feel your chest rise, and then be aware of your stomach and abdomen also pushing upwards as your lungs fill with air. When your lungs feel full, pause for a moment. Ideally, the hand on your abdomen will be higher than the one on your chest. Now, gradually let the air out from your stomach and abdomen first, then your chest. You should feel your muscles start to relax as you breathe out. Do this a few times during the day and again at night to help you relax before sleep.

Breathing is an important aspect of meditation, the state in which the mind is freed from its usual concerns. One analogy is that the mind in meditation is like a cloudless sky – the clouds being the clutter that obscures the blueness or mental clarity. A meditative state is one that is 'unclouded' by thoughts, feelings, etc., and you need to learn how to 'let go' of these thoughts. In meditation, the exhalation or 'out' breath signals the point of letting go of anxious thoughts. There are many books and CDs available telling you how to meditate, or you could join a meditation class to learn under expert guidance. Ask at your local library, adult education centre or Buddhist meditation centre.

Homeopathy

Homeopathy is a complementary medicine based on the idea that a substance that produces symptoms similar to those present in a disorder can be used, in greatly diluted form, to treat that disorder. It is the principle of treating like with like: so, for example, an onion makes the eyes stream, so use onion to treat a cold. There is some scientific basis to this particular remedy – we know that onion contains allicin and that allicin has both antibiotic and anti-viral properties. However, experts are divided as to the efficacy of homeopathy; some are convinced that it provides safe, natural and effective treatments for a number of conditions, others feel it has at best a placebo effect and can at worst delay the diagnosis of more serious illnesses. Homeopathy aims to treat the whole person as well as the individual symptoms, so the homeopath will ask a lot of questions about your general lifestyle and personality as well as your medical history. The idea is that a good knowledge of the individual enables the homeopath to select the remedy most likely to stimulate that person's own healing mechanisms. If you decide to try homeopathy, make sure you use a qualified and registered homeopath. Contact the Society of Homeopaths (see p. 111) to find a practitioner near you.

Acupuncture and acupressure

Acupuncture is a system of Chinese medicine that aims to stimulate the body's own healing responses by the use of fine needles inserted at strategic points around the body. Traditional Chinese philosophy teaches that our health is dependent on the body's natural energy – known as qi or chi – moving in a balanced way along meridians or channels beneath the skin. The flow of qi can be disturbed by physical, mental or emotional factors such as: injury, infection, poor nutrition, anxiety, stress or anger, fear or grief, weather conditions or hereditary factors. By inserting fine needles into the channels of energy, an acupuncturist can restore the balance, thus stimulating the body's healing process. Acupressure works in much the same way except that the therapist uses finger or hand pressure instead of needles. There is some evidence to suggest that these treatments are effective in treating insomnia, but experts say more research is needed.

Aromatherapy

The use of fragrant essential oils can have both psychological and physical effects, improving mood and promoting relaxation. Oils can be diluted in a 'carrier oil' and massaged into the skin, added to bathwater, inhaled neat or added to water and heated in an oil burner. Lavender oil is well known for its relaxation and sleep-inducing qualities, but there are other oils, clary sage or neroli for example, that may help. Essential oils should be always used with care, and it's best to check with a qualified aromatherapist before using them. To find a qualified aromatherapist, contact the International Federation of Professional Aromatherapists (details on p. 109).

Reflexology

Reflexology dates back to Ancient Egypt, India and China, but was introduced to the West in the early twentieth century as 'zone therapy' after it was noted that reflex areas on the feet and hands were linked to other areas and organs of the body within the same zone. This zone theory was developed into what is now known as reflexology, the idea that congestion or tension in any part of the foot is mirrored in the corresponding part of the body. A trained reflexologist can detect these subtle changes in the foot and, by applying massage or gentle pressure to specific points, can bring about change in the corresponding parts of the body. This action restores and balances the energy, qi or chi, within the body. Again, scientific research on the efficacy of reflexology is scant and of poor quality. However, anecdotal evidence suggests that it can be effective in treating a number of conditions, including insomnia, fatigue, stress and depression. There is no doubt that a foot massage is in itself relaxing, and many people find that they sleep very well after a reflexology treatment. Experts agree that while it can't be proved that reflexology works, it is unlikely to do any harm. Contact the Association of Reflexologists (see p. 107) to find a qualified therapist.

Light therapy

This is where a special lamp or light box is used to deliver a 'dose' of light at certain times in order to help regulate the internal body clock. During the hours of darkness the brain releases large amounts of melatonin, the hormone that is supposed to keep us asleep. When day breaks, light penetrates the brain via the retina, causing melatonin production to cease and stimulating the release of 'waking' and activity hormones. If the brain does not receive enough light – in the case of night workers, for example – the circadian rhythm or body clock is thrown off balance and the whole sleep pattern disrupted. Light therapy ensures that adequate light is delivered at the right time to help regulate the secretion of the sleep–wake hormones. Light therapy usually involves sitting in front of a light box for anything from 30 minutes to two hours a day, in one or two sessions. The density of light you need (measured as 'lux') and the length of exposure required will depend on your individual needs and response to the treatment, so there's a certain amount of trial and error involved. Because light boxes come in various shapes and sizes, you can pick something to suit your lifestyle and specific requirements. For more information on light boxes and how they work, have a look at <www.lumie.com> or see p. 109 for contact details. Light boxes are also used to treat Seasonal Affective Disorder (SAD), where those with the condition feel lethargic and depressed over the winter months because, it is thought, of the shortage of natural daylight.

Yoga

Yoga is a generic word meaning 'union'; it is often interpreted as the union of mind, body and soul, and when practised success-fully can provide perfect harmony and balance. There are different forms but Hatha yoga, the yoga of physical action, is most popular in the West and is the form practised in most Western yoga classes. It involves controlled stretching and breathing techniques, some meditation and some theory and philosophy. Practising yoga regu-larly can help improve your overall fitness and wellbeing as well as specifically improving flexibility, reducing stress and aiding relaxa-tion, all of which can lead to improved quality of sleep. To find out more about yoga or to find a teacher, contact the British Wheel of Yoga, the governing body for yoga in Great Britain (see p. 108).

Herbal medicines

There are so many herbal sleep remedies on the market that the choice can be bewildering. Some herbs can be taken in the form of teas – camomile, lemon balm and mint are all said to help promote drowsiness – while others can only be found as actual medicines. Many people are attracted to herbal remedies because they are 'natural', but this must not be confused with 'safe'; while the vast majority of herbal medicines are perfectly safe to take in accordance with the instructions, some remedies can be harmful if not taken correctly.

Nytol, the makers of a popular over-the-counter remedy (con-taining a sedating antihistamine), now make a herbal version of their remedy. Nytol Herbal contains five herbs known to have sedative properties: hops, wild lettuce, passiflora, dogwood Jamaica and pulsatilla. One of the most effective herbal remedies for stress, anxiety and insomnia is valerian. Try Sedonium, a standardized valerian extract, now licensed by the Medicines Control Agency for sleep disorders. The tablets contain the clinically proven dose of valerian, and the fact that the product is licensed means that it has undergone rigorous trials to test its efficacy.

Always remember that herbal remedies are medicines and, just as with conventional medicines, you should not take them if you are pregnant, suffer from a known medical condition or are taking any other conventional or herbal medicine without first checking with a registered herbalist and with your doctor or pharmacist. To find a registered herbalist near you, contact the National Institute of Medical Herbalists (see p. 110).

Quick reference guide to good sleep hygiene: ten top tips for a good night's kip

1 A warm (not hot) bath before bed can help you to relax, especially if you add a few drops of lavender oil to the water.
2 Sprinkle lavender oil on your pillow or buy a lavender spray 'pillow mister'.
3 Avoid alcohol, tobacco and caffeine.
4 Try a cup of camomile tea or a milky drink before bed.
5 If you get too hot, wear loose cotton nightclothes or none at all; if you suffer from cold feet, buy some bedsocks.
6 Use good quality cotton bedlinen.
7 Replace an old or worn-out mattress – buy the best you can afford.
8 Make sure the room is as dark as it can be. Fit blackout blinds if necessary.
9 If you are disturbed by noise, buy some earplugs. They won't block all environmental noise, but they should dull it enough for you to get some sleep.
10 Buy a thermometer and check the temperature of your bedroom. The ideal temperature is between 16 and 18 degrees Celsius (60 and 65 degrees Fahrenheit) – a bit chilly while you're getting undressed, but not once you've been in bed for a few minutes.

7

What your doctor can do

So far, this book has focused mainly on self-help for sleep difficulties, but in some cases you'll need more professional help. Depending on the underlying cause, there are a number of options available to your doctor. As we have seen, sleep disturbance can be linked with other medical conditions and it's important that this is investigated. It's possible that simply treating an underlying condition such as heartburn or back pain will make a considerable difference. If you're already being treated for a medical condition, it may be the medication itself that is the problem, so it's important to tell your doctor if you think this is the case – there may be a similar medicine that does not have this side effect. Other options include sleeping tablets or referral to a sleep clinic.

Sleeping tablets

In some cases, your doctor may suggest you take sleeping tablets, although this is usually considered as a last resort. If you are offered sleeping tablets, you should be aware of the pros and cons before making a decision.

When might sleeping tablets be prescribed?

Current advice is that sleeping tablets should only be prescribed for short periods when someone is suffering from severe insomnia, where the underlying cause is known, and where other treatment options have been considered. It is always preferable to treat the underlying cause, but in some cases, if the insomnia is causing extreme distress, sleeping tablets can be used to tide someone over until other treatment can be agreed. An example would be where someone cannot sleep after having been bereaved, or where someone is having difficulty sleeping after retiring from a job that involved night shifts. In both cases, sleeping tablets should be considered as a last resort and should only be prescribed for the briefest possible period.

The downside

There are several reasons why today's doctors are reluctant to prescribe sleeping pills. These include:

- Dependence – some types of sleeping pill cause dependence; in other words, they are addictive. This means that if you stop taking them suddenly, you are liable to experience withdrawal symptoms such as anxiety, shakiness, headaches, blurred vision, nausea, depression and many other unpleasant symptoms – including insomnia!
- Tolerance – this where your body becomes so used to the drug that it needs higher and higher doses to have the same effect.
- Drowsiness the next day – this is a problem with most sleeping tablets. It may affect your daily life if you need to drive or operate machinery.
- Risk of accident during the night – because sleeping tablets are designed to make you sleepy, there is a risk that you'll be disorientated, confused or clumsy if you get up in the night. Older people who take sleeping tablets have an increased risk of falls – it has been shown that the risk of hip fracture increases threefold in those taking temazepam.
- Side effects – there is a risk of unwanted side effects with all medicines, but sleeping tablets seem to have more than their fair share (see the next section), some of which can be quite debilitating. Always read the patient information leaflet that comes with your tablets.

Types of sleeping pill

In the past, doctors often prescribed barbiturates as a sleeping aid. They were very effective but the risk of dependence was high, as was the risk of death from overdose. Barbiturates are thought to have caused or contributed to the deaths, either deliberately or accidentally, of a number of famous people including Marilyn Monroe, Kenneth Williams, Elvis Presley and Jimmi Hendrix. These days, barbiturates are used mainly to treat epilepsy, although they are still occasionally prescribed for short periods to treat insomnia in the elderly.

Benzodiazepines

Benzodiazepines have been around since the 1960s and are now the most commonly used sleeping pills. They are only available on prescription and include: nitrazepam, flurazepam, loprazolam, lormetazepam and temazepam.

Possible side effects

Benzodiazepines all have similar side effects. The most common are: drowsiness and light-headedness the next day, confusion and unsteadiness (especially in the elderly), forgetfulness, muscle weakness, dependence and difficulties with withdrawal.

Less common side effects include: headaches, stomach upsets, low blood pressure, joint pain, skin rashes, change in libido, incontinence and difficulty urinating. In a few people, the drugs cause excitability and even aggressive or hostile behaviour.

Nitrazepam and flurazepam are fairly long-acting and therefore are more likely to give a 'hangover effect' the next day. Loprazolam, lormetazepam and temazepam are short-acting and therefore less likely to cause a hangover effect; they are, however, more likely to cause withdrawal problems.

Z drugs

These are more recently introduced than the benzodiazepines, but although they are different drugs they act in a similar way and work on the same brain receptors. They are only available on prescription and include: zolpidem, zopiclone and zaleplon.

Possible side effects

The Z drugs are all short-acting and have little or no hangover effect. Like the benzodiazepines, they are associated with dependence and can cause withdrawal problems, so they should be given at the lowest effective dose and for the shortest possible time. Zolpidem and zopiclone should only be used for a maximum of four weeks, and the manufacturers of zaleplon recommend a maximum of two weeks.

- Zolpidem (Stilnoct) – diarrhoea, nausea, vomiting, dizziness, headaches, daytime drowsiness, weakness, memory problems, nightmares, reduced alertness, confusion, unsteadiness, double vision, upset stomach, changes in libido, skin rashes, depression, excitability or hostility, dependence.
- Zopiclone (Zimovane) – mild bitter or metallic after-taste, nausea, vomiting, dizziness, headache, upset stomach, drowsiness and dry mouth. More rarely: irritability, aggressiveness, confusion, depression, memory problems, nightmares, skin rashes, light-headedness and loss of coordination.
- Zaleplon (Sonata) – memory loss, tingling sensations, drowsiness, loss of energy. More rarely: nausea, loss of appetite, feeling weak, hypoaesthesia (reduced sensation), sensitivity to light, unsteadiness, confusion, loss of concentration, apathy, feeling detached from things, depression, dizziness, hallucinations, slurred speech, visual disturbances, excitability or hostility. Very rarely: severe allergic reactions.

Antihistamines

Although antihistamines are primarily used to treat allergic reactions in conditions such as hay fever, they are sometimes used as a sleeping aid owing to their main side effect – drowsiness. Antihistamine is the active ingredient in a number of sleeping medicines that you can buy without a prescription. Even though they're not as powerful as the prescription drugs, they may cause a hangover effect and residual drowsiness in the morning.

Possible side effects

These include dizziness, restlessness, headaches, nightmares, tiredness and disorientation. Occasionally, especially in older people: blurred vision, dry mouth, urine retention, confusion and excitability. More rarely: loss of appetite, stomach discomfort, palpitations, low blood pressure, disturbances of heart rhythm, shaking, muscle spasms, tic-like movements, blood disorders and sensitivity to sunlight. If you're taking any other medication or are not sure whether an antihistamine is suitable, check with the pharmacist before buying.

Coming off sleeping pills

The effects of sleeping pills vary from person to person, and your level of tolerance and risk of dependence will also vary, but it is possible to become addicted to sleeping pills in as little as two weeks. If you have been taking sleeping pills every night, or almost every night, for two weeks or longer, you should talk to your doctor about weaning yourself off them. The longer you've been taking them, the more difficult this can be and the more anxious you're likely to be about coping without them. If you just stop taking your pills, you're more likely to experience withdrawal symptoms and this makes coming off them even more difficult.

Most doctors will advise you to taper off, gradually reducing the dosage. Theoretically, the slower you taper off, the milder the withdrawal symptoms. You can cut even quite small tablets with a scalpel or razor blade, so it's possible to reduce your dose very gradually. Any reduction in dose is going to be a shock to your system, so reduce by small amounts – an eighth at a time if possible – and leave at least three or four days in between reductions to allow your body to readjust. Always do this with the supervision of your doctor. Sheldon Press also publishes a book on how to withdraw from this kind of drug – *Tranquillizers and Antidepressants: When to Start Them, How to Stop,* by Professor Malcolm Lader, Emeritus Professor of Clinical Psychopharmacology, King's College London.

You will probably be worried that you won't be able to sleep at all if you stop taking the sleeping pills, and sometimes just the anxiety itself can keep you awake. While you're weaning yourself off these drugs, make sure you are scrupulous about 'sleep hygiene'; be aware of the things that can help you sleep, and of those that can stop you from sleeping. See Chapter 6 for lots of advice on how to get a good night's sleep without taking sleeping pills.

Your doctor should only have prescribed sleeping pills if your insomnia was severe. Often, this is the result of a bereavement or some other trauma in your life. If this is the case, you may need some counselling to help you to come to terms with what has happened. Talk to your doctor about this, and he or she may be able to refer you. Or you could seek this out yourself. See the Useful addresses section (p. 107) for details of appropriate organizations.

Sleep clinics

If your doctor is unsure what's causing the problem, or if he or she suspects you may have sleep apnoea, a referral to a sleep clinic may be in order. These clinics may be found within ordinary hospitals or they may be completely separate. They may be referred to as sleep clinics, sleep labs or sleep disorder centres.

What happens at a sleep clinic?

Before attending your initial appointment, you may be asked to fill in a detailed sleep questionnaire and/or to keep a sleep diary (see p. 62). At the appointment, you'll see a specialist in sleep disorders or possibly an ear, nose and throat (ENT) specialist. ENT surgeons often have a special interest in sleep disorders, and in particular snoring and sleep apnoea. Many of the UK's sleep clinics focus on snoring and sleep apnoea, although there are some that deal with general sleep disorders. The specialist will take a full medical history and ask you specifically about your sleep patterns, before carrying out an assessment to see how serious the difficulty is and decide whether you need further treatment.

In order for the situation to be assessed, you will probably need to undertake a simple sleep study such as a pulse oximetry, which measures your heart rate and blood oxygen levels. This may be done at the hospital or sleep centre, or you may be asked to carry it out at home using a device that you attach to your finger or one that you wear like a wristwatch. Pulse oximetry is often used to diagnose breathing-related sleep disorders such as sleep apnoea. Actigraphy is another type of study that you may be asked to carry out at home, particularly if the doctor suspects you may have restless legs syndrome (see p. 44). The study measures levels of movement and involves wearing a movement monitor, also resembling a wristwatch, on your arm or leg for a few days and nights at home. Sometimes the results of these studies are not conclusive and a full overnight polysomnogram (PSG) will be recommended. This involves an overnight stay at the hospital or sleep centre, and includes the following tests:

- electro-encephalography (EEG) – brain-wave monitoring;
- electromyography (EMG) – muscle-tone monitoring;

- recording thoracic–abdominal movements – chest and abdomen movements;
- recording oro-nasal flow – mouth and nose air flow;
- pulse oximetry – heart rate and blood oxygen-level monitoring;
- electrocardiography (ECG) – heart monitoring.

It is a very detailed study and can help to diagnose a range of sleep disorders, including sleep apnoea, restless legs syndrome and parasomnias such as narcolepsy and sleepwalking.

A night in the sleep clinic

If you're referred for an overnight stay, you should be given detailed instructions and a good idea of what to expect. Different centres will have different admissions procedures, but usually you'll be asked to arrive late in the afternoon, or possibly after your evening meal (some centres provide supper, others only offer breakfast the following morning). You'll need your own nightclothes and toiletries, and probably your own towel. It's also a good idea to take some reading matter. Don't forget any medications you usually take, and make sure you show these to the staff.

Usually you'll follow an admissions procedure where more details will be taken, then you'll be shown to your room. Rooms in sleep clinics are not quite five-star hotel standard, but they're usually very comfortable with a bed, chair and television. Private clinics may be slightly more luxurious. Once you're settled in your room, you can read or watch television before performing your usual bedtime ablutions and changing into your night things, probably a little earlier than usual. The sleep technician will then come along and attach various electrodes and sensors to different parts of your body to record your temperature, heart rate, movements and so on. This may feel strange and inconvenient, but none of it will cause discomfort. The electrodes are attached with glue (which is easily removed the following morning) to your scalp and face in order to measure brainwaves, chin muscle tone and eye movements. There is no need to shave off any hair tc do this. Movement sensors will be attached to your legs to check muscle activity and a chest band will be used to detect breathing movements such as the rise and fall of your ribcage. Electrodes may also be attached to the chest in order to monitor the heart. There may be sensors attached to the nose and below the mouth, to measure air-flow, and a sensor attached to a finger to measure the blood oxygen levels. You may also be asked to wear a microphone around your neck to record snoring, or there may be other sound or video recording equipment in the room.

You'll then be asked to tell the staff when you're ready to settle for the night, and left to read or whatever until you're ready to go to sleep. When you're ready the technician will come along and hook up all the various wires to a junction box, situated near the head of the bed so that you can turn over if you need to. The technician will check that everything is properly connected and show you which button or buzzer to press if you need to use the loo in the night (someone will come along to unhook you so you can walk to the lavatory), then you can settle down to sleep. You probably think it would be virtually impossible to sleep with all these wires attached, but many people sleep surprisingly well at the sleep clinic – even when they're suffering from insomnia!

In the morning, usually between 6 and 7 a.m., the monitoring equipment will be disconnected and the data collected and passed for analysis. The analysis will take some time and you won't receive the full results for a few days or even longer. The person analysing the results will look with particular interest at:

- sleep latency – how long it took you to fall asleep;
- sleep efficiency – how long you were actually asleep compared with how long you were lying in bed with your eyes closed;
- sleep stages – how long you spent in light, deep and REM sleep;
- breathing irregularities like apnoea;
- 'arousals' – these are indicated by a sudden shift in the brain-wave activity, which could be due to leg movements, environmental conditions, breathing issues, etc.;
- heart rhythm abnormalities;
- body position during sleep;
- leg movement patterns;
- oxygen saturation.

When you're dressed and have had breakfast, you'll be able to go home. Staff may discuss your preliminary results with you briefly, but it's more likely that this will happen some time after your visit. When all the information has been analysed, you'll be given another appointment at which the doctor will talk you through the results and recommend treatment, if appropriate, or maybe further testing.

Yvonne

Yvonne, 74, spent a night in a sleep clinic last year to check whether she was suffering from sleep apnoea.

> I often felt tired during the day, but I put it down to getting older. Then I read something about sleep apnoea and I remembered that my husband used to say that I sometimes seemed to stop breathing when I was asleep. I mentioned this to my GP, who referred me to a specialist. But when I told the specialist that I would often wake up with a pain in my hip, which could only be relieved by getting up and walking about, he said it could be restless legs syndrome, and referred me to the sleep clinic in St Thomas's Hospital in London.
>
> When I arrived for my night's stay at the clinic, a nurse weighed me, took my blood pressure and so on, and showed me the large comfortable room where I would sleep and also the technician's room, which was full of computers. She explained that I would be connected to a monitoring system that would record my sleep patterns on these computers. After having a meal in the hospital restaurant, I showered and prepared for bed; they told me not to use any body lotions or hair conditioner as these might interfere with the monitoring. Then the technician came in and stuck small discs on various parts of my body, ready to be connected up to the monitor before I went to sleep. It was quite early in the evening, so I spent some time looking out at the River Thames, then I sat in a small sitting room reading for a while before going back to my room. When I was ready to settle down, the nurse came in and attached each of the discs to wires, which she connected to a monitor. She said I should ring the bell if I wanted to get up during the night and someone would come and disconnect me. I wondered how I would sleep, but the bed was very comfortable, and after reading briefly I soon dropped off. I woke up a few times and got up twice to go to the toilet. In the morning, after I was disconnected, the technician asked if I was always that restless. I said yes, I was. I didn't know at that point that it was unusual to have to get up and remake the bed two or three times a night!

When I attended the follow-up appointment, the doctor told me that I didn't have sleep apnoea but I did have RLS. He prescribed an anti-convulsive medicine, and since then I've slept much better and I no longer have to remake the bed during the night!

Cognitive behaviour therapy (CBT)

This is becoming an increasingly popular method of treating long-term insomnia, and it may be recommended by your family doctor, or possibly by the sleep clinic. CBT works on the principle that negative thought-patterns have been learned over time, and that they can be 'unlearned' and replaced with more healthy, positive thoughts. The treatment aims to use thoughts (cognitive) to change actions (behaviour).

A therapist treating someone with insomnia will teach that person how to recognize, challenge and change the negative ways of thinking that may be keeping him or her awake. For example, many insomniacs worry excessively about not being able to sleep, causing a stress response that actually stops them from dropping off. The CBT therapist can help by educating the person about the nature and function of sleep, average sleep needs and better sleep hygiene. He or she might teach that person how to 'let go' of wakefulness rather than worry about not being able to go to sleep – the insomniac should never 'try' to go to sleep. The therapist might also suggest setting aside half an hour during the day specifically for worrying; this helps to remove or at least reduce the tendency to worry at night. It might also be helpful to write down the worries – sometimes things don't seem as bad when you see them on paper. The therapist may offer other techniques for de-cluttering your mind and coping with night-time worry. One such method is to imagine, with your eyes closed, that your worry is a balloon; imagine it floating up into the air, then mentally burst it. Worry gone!

Insomniacs often have a distorted idea of how badly they sleep. It's not uncommon for them to say they haven't slept at all, or they didn't drop off until five and then woke again at seven. In fact, if you measure their sleep, you see they slept for four or five hours. This may be because, when you can't sleep, it can *feel* as though you've been awake all night. CBT can help people to understand that their perceptions may not be quite accurate.

The combination of changing negative, wakefulness-inducing thought patterns and improving daily sleep hygiene can make a big difference, even to those who have chronic insomnia. Ideally, you will be referred to a therapist who specializes in sleep matters, but more general CBT should help, and it's even something you can teach yourself to a certain extent – see Further reading, p. 112.

8

Other sleep disorders in adults

Up until now, this book has concentrated on the difficulties caused by not being able to get to sleep, early waking and poor quality sleep, all of which we tend to refer to as insomnia. Sometimes our sleep is disturbed by other sleep disorders, some of which can have a serious effect on a person's health and wellbeing and can also affect his or her family.

Nightmares

Nightmares are extended disturbing and frightening dreams where we feel under threat. The threat can be to ourselves or to our loved ones and may pertain to physical safety or survival, emotional wellbeing, security or self-esteem. On waking, the nightmare is still very vivid and the whole thing recalled in detail. We've all suffered nightmares at some point, and children tend to have them more frequently than adults – there's more about children's sleep difficulties in Chapter 9. Half of all adults say they have the occasional nightmare, and around 1 per cent of the population has a nightmare every week. Women report two to four nightmares for every one nightmare reported by men. What we don't know is whether men and women actually experience different rates of nightmares, or whether women are simply more likely to report them. In fact, most estimates of adult prevalence of nightmares are unreliable, because the definition of what constitutes a nightmare varies from person to person, as does the ability to recall dreams the following morning.

It is thought that nightmares in adults are fairly rare. They are usually unpleasant at the time and immediately afterwards, but not enough of a problem to disturb sleep on a regular basis. Exceptions include people suffering from Post-Traumatic Stress Disorder (PTSD), Nightmare Disorder, drug or alcohol addiction or drug or alcohol withdrawal. PTSD can arise after any traumatic experience and involves flashbacks – where the experience is relived or replayed like a film – and nightmares, where the experience may be revisited as it happened or mutated into something equally terrifying. If you think you may be suffering from PTSD, talk to your doctor – there are a number of psychological treatments for PTSD, and according to the Centre for Anxiety Disorders and Trauma (see p. 108 for contact details) these are usually effective without additional medication.

Laura

Laura, 32, began to suffer terrible nightmares after her baby was born by emergency caesarean section. It was only when she discovered that she was suffering from Post-Traumatic Stress Disorder that she was able to address the cause of her symptoms.

> My daughter's birth was a terrifying experience. I knew there was something wrong halfway through my labour but no-one believed me, then the baby went into distress and suddenly everyone was shouting and dashing around. They rushed me to theatre and, thank God, Polly was delivered safely. But within days, I started to suffer flashbacks and nightmares about the birth. It was like a film running in my head. There was no escape, whether I was awake or asleep. I just kept seeing it happen all over again – them lifting me onto the trolley, it hitting the walls as they rushed me to theatre, all their voices raised in panic.
>
> During the first months of Polly's life, I was exhausted, partly from caring for a new baby but also because I was hardly sleeping. The worst thing was that I felt guilty: after all, millions of women give birth every day – why had I found it such a problem?
>
> Eventually, I mentioned it to my health visitor. She was fantastic; she said it sounded like I was suffering from PTSD and suggested I ask my doctor about some counselling. Just the fact that she acknowledged my feelings really helped, and in the end I didn't need counselling as such. At first I'd thought I was the only woman who'd been traumatized by childbirth. But then I found others through baby websites. Discussing the experience with women who understand has really helped. Gradually, once I'd started really talking about it, the nightmares began to diminish, disappearing completely by Polly's first birthday. These days I sleep much better, and only wake up when Polly decides she wants to play games at two in the morning!

Nightmare Disorder, where someone experiences frequent night-mares without any of the usual causes (PTSD, drug or alcohol abuse or withdrawal) is rare in adults, but not unheard of. The disorder is only diagnosed when other causes have been ruled out and when the nightmares are having a serious impact on the person's life. Someone who suffers from frequent nightmares may develop insomnia as a result. This may be due to a reluctance, which may or may not be conscious, to go to sleep in case the nightmares return; it may be due to the frequent waking that may accompany night-mares; or it may be because you have begun to associate sleep with fear and distress. Whatever the cause of your nightmares, if they are disturbing your sleep on a regular basis, talk to your doctor – there may be help available.

Night terrors

Night terrors, which occur during deep sleep, are completely dif-ferent from nightmares. They are not exactly bad dreams but sudden, terrifying sensations with fleeting mental images that shock the sleeper into immediate wakefulness. During a night terror, the sleeper's heart rate quickens and he or she may shout or appear in distress, perhaps shaking and thrashing about. In some cases, people in the midst of a night terror can thrash around so violently as to cause injury to themselves or to someone else. Night terrors were once thought to occur only in children, but we now know that, although it's fairly rare, adults can suffer from them as well. Night terrors are common in children and are perfectly normal, but in adults they could indicate an underlying psychological or neuro-logical cause that needs to be investigated, so if you think you may be experiencing night terrors, talk to your doctor about this. For a more detailed look at night terrors in children, see p. 101.

Sleepwalking

Again, this disorder is more common in children; however, a 2006 study by the hotel chain Travelodge indicated that one in ten adults is a regular sleepwalker. Travelodge commissioned the study after an increase in the number of guests sleepwalking in hotels. One hotel reported three separate incidents of guests walking into reception while still asleep – and stark naked!

Sleepwalking occurs during deep sleep and may begin quite abruptly. The sleeper sits up in bed, then gets up and wanders around the room with a blank expression on his or her face. Sometimes the movements are clumsy and purposeless (although sleepwalkers do seem to able negotiate furniture fairly well), sometimes they are quite complex – there are reports of people eating, drinking, playing a musical instrument or even driving or trying to make a telephone call while still fast asleep. Often the only clue that the person is asleep is that what he or she says is incoherent. There have been some cases where sleepwalking has been used as a defence when someone has committed a crime. Recently, a young man with a history of sleepwalking was found not guilty of rape after a jury heard a sleep expert explain that it was possible for someone to carry out such an act while asleep, with no awareness of what he was doing, or any recollection afterwards.

We don't really know why people sleepwalk, but it is thought that stress, alcohol, some medications and sleep deprivation may trigger a bout of sleepwalking. There is also a link between night terrors and sleepwalking. Adults with a history of sleepwalking may find that it recurs at times of stress or sleep deprivation. The biggest danger to the sleepwalker is injury, with many sleepwalkers suffering cuts, bruises and even broken bones. Contrary to popular belief, it is not dangerous to wake a sleepwalker; however, he or she is likely to be quite deeply asleep and therefore difficult to wake and disoriented on waking, so the best option is to avoid this by simply guiding the person back to bed.

Narcolepsy

Narcolepsy is a neurological condition where there is a fault in the mechanism of the brain that controls the sleep–wake cycle. This manifests as excessive daytime sleepiness, which can result in someone falling asleep suddenly and at inappropriate times. Cataplexy, a sudden loss of muscle control, often triggered by strong emotions such as anger, amusement, shock or excitement, may also be present. Cataplexy is only found in narcolepsy, so the presence of this symptom makes diagnosis easier. Narcolepsy is thought to be relatively rare, although it is also significantly under-reported, so it is difficult to estimate how many people are affected.

The condition was first recognized in the late nineteenth century, but it wasn't until a hundred years later that we began to understand narcolepsy and what may cause it. A neurotransmitter called orexin (also known as hypocretin) is thought to play an important role in the control of the sleep–wake cycle. At the end of the twentieth century, scientists found that mice that couldn't make orexin in their brains developed narcolepsy; at around the same time, dogs with narcolepsy were found to have a faulty orexin receptor. The implications were clear, and more investigations followed. Sure enough, in humans with narcolepsy, the levels of orexin were found to be low or even undetectable in the brain and spinal fluid, and the nerves containing orexin had degenerated. However, research is still in its early stages and is ongoing. The condition tends to run in families, and studies suggest that you're up to 50 times more likely to develop narcolepsy if you have a close relative with the condition. The age of onset is usually adolescence or early adulthood, although it can develop much later in some people.

The symptoms of narcolepsy can be very distressing. The level of sleepiness during the day can be so high that the individual can be rendered incapable of performing even routine tasks competently. When the compulsion to sleep is really strong, the person may appear drunk, and may fall asleep involuntarily and very suddenly. This could clearly be devastating if someone was in the middle of bathing a baby, frying chips or painting the ceiling. He or she may also experience 'micro-sleeps'. This is where the person sleeps for 20–30 seconds without being aware of it. This can be embarrassing if, for example, it happens in mid-conversation; the narcoleptic drifts into a micro-sleep and comes out of it, completely unaware and still at the point of conversation where he or she left it. The talk has moved on and everyone is staring open-mouthed at the poor narcoleptic, whose conversation is now out of synch.

The other major symptom, cataplexy, can be so mild as to cause only a slight slackening of the facial muscles, or so severe that the person collapses on the floor. Speech may be slurred and eyesight affected, but hearing and awareness remain unimpaired. The attacks usually last for a few minutes, after which things either return to normal or leave the individual needing a long sleep. An attack is more likely when the person is tired. Other symptoms include temporary paralysis, hallucinations or nightmares on falling asleep or on waking, short periods of 'trance-like' behaviour and frequent night waking accompanied by a rapid heartbeat. Not everyone with narcolepsy will experience all of these symptoms.

If you think you may have narcolepsy, talk to your doctor. He or she may refer you to a specialist for further investigations. Narcolepsy cannot be cured at present, but the symptoms can often be controlled by making lifestyle changes, and in most cases this should be tried before considering medication. Try, for example,

- sticking to regular times for getting up and going to bed;
- avoiding heavy meals and too much alcohol;
- avoiding jobs where shift work is required, or that involve long periods of intense concentration and physical immobility;
- recognizing periods of low alertness and establishing a routine of regular naps, physical activity and breaks in the open air to combat sleepiness;
- recognizing and avoiding situations that are likely to trigger an attack of cataplexy.

Taking these steps will hopefully eliminate or reduce the need for medication. However, if the sleepiness is severe, it may be treated with stimulant drugs such as amphetamine, which, although it's often thought of as a 'street drug', is licensed for the treatment of narcolepsy. Cataplexy can be treated with antidepressants – this is not because people with the condition are necessarily depressed, but because one of the side effects of this type of medication is to inhibit the neurological pathways that cause cataplexy.

If you are diagnosed with narcolepsy you must inform the DVLA. Failure to do so is a criminal offence and you could be fined up to £1,000, as well as finding your insurance cover invalidated. Usually, the DVLA will issue a temporary licence, reassessed every one, two or three years, as long as your doctor can satisfy the DVLA that your condition is adequately controlled by treatment.

Hypersomnia

This is when somebody sleeps very deeply or for prolonged periods, and may have extreme difficulty in waking up. The term is also used to describe excessive sleepiness like that associated with narcolepsy, where other symptoms such as cataplexy or sleep paralysis may be present. Hypersomnia is also a symptom of depression (as is insomnia), and it may be also a feature of the depressive phases of bi-polar disorder. Someone with hypersomnia can sleep for 12 hours a night and still feel sleepy during the day. If there appears to be no underlying cause, the condition is described as 'idiopathic hypersomnia'. There is no specific treatment for the condition but, as with narcolepsy, lifestyle changes and improved sleep hygiene may help.

Klein-Levin Syndrome

The symptoms of this rare neurological disorder include recurring episodes of hypersomnia and changes in the person's usual behaviour. At the onset of an episode he (the condition primarily affects males aged 10–25) becomes drowsy, either progressively or suddenly, and sleeps for most of the day and night, waking only to perform essential functions such as eating, drinking or using the lavatory. When awake, he may seem confused, disorientated, lethargic and apathetic. People with this syndrome may have difficulty focusing and find they are hypersensitive to noise and light. In some cases, they experience powerful food cravings and exhibit hypersexual behaviour. It is thought that the symptoms may be related to malfunction of the hypothalamus, the part of the brain that controls appetite and sleep. Episodes may occur several times a year. There is no treatment at present and in most cases the symptoms disappear with advancing age, but the condition can be extremely distressing in the meantime.

Sleep paralysis

This can happen as you're falling asleep or just as you wake up; as the name suggests, you suddenly find yourself completely unable to move. It can last for anything from a few seconds to a few minutes, which can be very frightening if you don't know what's happening. Sleep paralysis occurs because of a mistiming between the systems that control the normal muscle paralysis of REM sleep and those that control wakefulness. So, in other words, the paralysis is normal – it's the result of hormones released by the body to prevent us from acting out our dreams – but we're usually unaware of it because we're asleep when it occurs. Most of the muscles that control breathing are unaffected, but some may be, and this may cause feelings of suffocation. Some people also experience visual and auditory hallucinations, along with a powerful sense of fear or impending death; if these accompany the sensation of an oppressive weight on the chest, making breathing difficult, you can see how you might seriously wonder if you are being attacked by some sort of demon! In fact, the condition is sometimes known as 'old hag syndrome', from the superstitious belief that a witch sits on or 'rides' the chest of those affected, rendering them immobile.

James

James, 24, had recently moved into a new flat when he experienced an episode of sleep paralysis, something he'd never heard of at the time.

> The flat was in an old Victorian house and my flatmates and I had joked when we moved in that it might be haunted. Then one night I woke to feel this heavy weight on my chest. I couldn't breathe, and I couldn't move. I could hear my heart beating and I remember thinking, *this can't be happening – I must be dreaming*. But I knew I was awake. Eventually, I managed to force my head to the side so that I was facing the door. I tried to call out to my flatmates, but I could only make a tiny sound low down in my throat. That was the most terrifying thing of all – trying to shout for help, but finding no sound would come out. It was like a waking nightmare. I didn't tell anyone for ages in case they thought I'd lost the plot. But then I mentioned it to my mum and it turned out she'd just heard something on the radio about sleep paralysis and she recognized it immediately. It hasn't happened again so far, but if it does I don't think I'll be as scared, now I know that it's not some creature of the night come to get me!

Like James, many people are reluctant to tell anyone about the experience for fear of being labelled mentally ill, but sleep paralysis is thought to be quite common – around half of the population will experience it at least once. It can occur at any age, but is more common in people under 30. We know very little about what causes sleep paralysis, but sleep disturbance and deprivation may be a factor; in fact the condition is often associated with narcolepsy (see p. 92) and is sometimes seen in sleep apnoea (p. 51).

Although unpleasant, the condition is not harmful, and most of those affected, once they know what is happening, feel less frightened by the episodes and find they can allow themselves to simply 'rest' into the paralysis and wait until it passes. You may be able to bring yourself out of the paralysis by attempting to breathe calmly and trying to move small body parts such as your eyelids, fingers or toes. You may find the Sleep Paralysis Information Service helpful. The organization was set up by those with the condition to raise awareness and provide information on this little talked-about condition. Visit their website at <www.spis.org.uk>.

9

Sleep difficulties in children

A wakeful child is often a major cause of adult sleep disturbance. If you are a new parent, you will have probably expected a certain number of sleepless nights, but may still be reeling from the reality of the profoundly altered sleep pattern that comes with your bundle of joy. And if your children have been sleeping through the night for some time, it can be quite a shock to find you have returned to those disturbed nights you thought were all in the past. The first step is to try and establish why your child is not sleeping, and from there you can look at the best options to help him or her (and therefore yourself) to get a good night's sleep.

Lack of routine

As we have seen, a bedtime routine is important for all of us, but for babies and young children it's even more so. How to establish a bedtime routine for a very young baby is a subject for a book in itself, and indeed there are many good books available. If you are struggling to cope with settling your new baby, ask your midwife, health visitor and other mums to recommend books they've found helpful, or for any tips and advice that might be useful. In the very early days, it's often a case of just making sure you sleep when the baby sleeps so that you have enough energy to care for him or her. As your baby gets older, however, you will be able to establish a routine. There may be lapses and it may take some time before you can really see that it's working, but the effort will pay off in the end.

Getting them off to bed

After the evening meal, keep activities fairly low key – now is not the time for a rough-and-tumble session. Try to establish a regular pattern: perhaps have a last snack or drink, brush teeth, bath, then pyjamas on and into bed for a story, music tape or, for older kids, half an hour's reading time. It's worth warning them in advance: if they're in the middle of an interesting game when Big Bad Mum tells them to stop and put everything away because it's time to go to bed, they're likely to resist. If bedtime is 7.30, for example, tell them about an hour beforehand that it's coming up. Then at 7 p.m. tell them they have 15 minutes' playing time left before they have to start getting ready for bed. At 7.15, it's time to get washed, brush teeth and change into their pyjamas, then at 7.30 it's into their bedrooms for a story or whatever. Remind them that the quicker they do this, the more time they'll have before lights out. You could even make a game out of getting ready quickly. Try setting a kitchen timer for each task: say, five minutes for a wash, 15 for a bath, one for getting into pyjamas, and so on.

If there's any more than about 18 months between them, it might be an idea to let the older one stay up a little later. Younger children will complain, but they'll get used to it, especially if you read them a story while their older sibling is still in the living room.

Keeping them there

Make sure that once they're in bed, there's no reason to get up again.

- If they're likely to want a drink of water, put one on the bedside table.
- Make sure they've been to the loo.
- Try to keep the bedroom at a comfortable temperature – if it's too warm or too cold, they'll find it difficult to settle.
- Make sure any favourite teddies or scraps of blanket are to hand.
- If they're afraid of the dark, leave the landing light on or give them a night light.
- If they insist there's a monster under the bed, tell them that monsters only exist in stories. Don't make a big deal of checking under the bed – you'll reinforce the fear – but show them there's

nothing there if really necessary. Get them to help you make up a story about a nice, kind, funny monster.

Nightmares

We all have nightmares occasionally (see p. 89) and the experience is unpleasant for all of us. For children, however, they can be especially frightening. Dreaming occurs during the phase known as REM sleep (see p. 4). Periods of REM sleep tend to get longer as the night progresses and so nightmares are more likely to occur in the second half of the night, by which time you're likely to be asleep. This means you may not immediately hear your child crying and may take a while to reach him or her. If your child has nightmares regularly, it may be worth installing a baby alarm so you can hear any crying straight away. It's also an idea to leave the landing light on so your child is able to get to you quickly if need be.

We know that daytime events often feature in our dreams, and a distressing or traumatic experience could well trigger nightmares in your child, as can disturbing news broadcasts or footage of tragic or disastrous events. Unfortunately, we can't protect our children from all life's horrors, but you can reduce the risk of nightmares. If something awful has happened in the world:

- Reassure your child that he or she is safe. Make it clear that, while these terrible things do happen, they are rare occurrences and that's why they are reported on the news.
- Avoid over-exposure to the media – don't let children watch distressing footage over and over again. Even if you feel you want to be glued to the screen to keep up with what is happening, make sure that it's not the only television your children see before going to bed.
- Answer their questions honestly, but keep the information age-appropriate.
- Encourage them to talk or draw pictures about their feelings.

Other triggers can be scary books or films, or irrational fears, such as a fear of the dark. This is very common in children, who may imagine monsters lurking in the shadows. Making them sleep in the dark to overcome their fear could have the opposite effect, triggering more nightmares or long-term anxiety. Leave the landing light on if you can, or buy a nightlight for their bedroom. Even a neon plug light provides a reassuring glow.

When they've had a nightmare they'll be upset and disorientated, so try and establish a sense of familiarity and security as soon as possible. Put the light on, make sure they have their favourite teddy or blanket and talk soothingly as they snuggle down again. Try giving them a fresh pillow to help have 'nice dreams'. As they get older, teach them a 'bad dream drill' so they can learn to cope on their own – light on, look around, cuddle teddy, snuggle down. Do this with them at first to help build their confidence. Most children learn to cope with the odd bad dream. If nightmares persist, however, try to find out if there's a reason you're not aware of. Is there something your child is worried or anxious about? Is everything all right at school? If you're still worried, or if your child continues to have difficulty going to sleep because of worries about nightmares, talk to your health visitor or doctor.

Night terrors

Night terrors (see p. 91) are very different from nightmares and require a different response. Unlike nightmares, night terrors usually occur in the first part of the night. While a nightmare usually consists of a frightening narrative, the night terror is more of a sensation or a brief image. The child may scream uncontrollably, sit up in bed or even get up and walk or run around, apparently awake and in extreme terror. In fact, the child is asleep and is likely to remain so throughout the duration of the night terror. As a parent, it's very upsetting to see your child apparently in such distress and your instinct will be to try and offer comfort. However, waking a child in the middle of a night terror may frighten him, making him lash out and appear even more terrified. All you can do is to wait in the room to make sure your child doesn't hurt himself. Night terrors are quite common in children, and are far more distressing for the parent than the child, who is unlikely to even remember the incident in the morning.

Sleepwalking

Sleepwalking is also common in childhood and is usually nothing to worry about. It may happen for no reason at all, or it can be triggered by illness, stress or lack of sleep. The sleepwalking child remains asleep although his or her eyes are open. Some children wander around slowly, apparently calm, with a glassy stare; others rush about in an agitated state. Eventually, the child may lie down (back in bed or somewhere else) and fall into a deeper sleep, or may wake up and describe a feeling of danger. It is not dangerous to wake children who are sleepwalking, but it could frighten or disorientate them. If possible, guide your child gently back to bed. If he or she doesn't remember the episode, there's not much point in mentioning it. If the child does remember, reassure her that sleepwalking is normal, quite common and that she'll probably grow out of it.

If the sleepwalking happens frequently, you could try using a technique known as 'scheduled waking', which can help some children. If the sleepwalking occurs at a similar time during the night, try waking your child about 15 minutes before the episode is due and repeat this every night for up to a month. Drugs can be used if sleepwalking is extremely disruptive or distressing, and where other measures have failed, but they would usually only be used as a last resort and for a short time.

Bedwetting

At around three and a half to four, most children start to wake up when they have a full bladder. However, children develop this skill at different rates, and a few may not achieve it until their teens. In the UK, one in six five-year-olds and around half a million children between the ages of six and 16 still wet the bed. Sometimes it may happen two or three times a night, meaning severe disruption to sleep for both you and your child.

First, check there's no practical cause – is your child avoiding that last trip to the loo for some reason? Could the thought of crossing a dark landing be too alarming for a visit to the bathroom during the night? See your doctor to make sure your child doesn't have a urine infection – an infection that causes pain on urinating can cause a child to hold on for too long or to try and avoid weeing altogether. If there's no obvious cause and your child is wetting the bed most nights, you may need professional help through an enuresis clinic. Talk to your doctor or health visitor about this. The clinic will assess each child individually before suggesting treatment, which may include an alarm, 'star charts' (depending on age) or medication to reduce the amount of urine produced at night. Treatment is usually successful, though it may take months or, in some cases, years.

In the meantime, make your life easier by making up the bed in layers, each with a waterproof sheet in between, and having spare nightclothes for your child easily to hand. That way, you can whip off the wet sheet and waterproof and put your child straight back into a dry bed, knowing that if he or she wets again there's another waterproof sheet underneath. Then you can bundle everything up, chuck it in the bath and crawl back into bed before you've really woken up. You could keep a pack of baby-wipes handy to give your child a quick clean up, or you could just leave it until the morning. If you use a top sheet as well as a duvet, you've more chance of keeping the duvet dry. If that doesn't work, use washable blankets until your child is dry.

Even if you do make life easier with the 'layer' system, having to get up two or three times a night to change wet sheets can be very trying, not to mention the pile of washing you have to do, but try not to be cross with your child. Children who wet the bed have to cope with considerable discomfort, sleep deprivation and embarrassment, and they are highly unlikely to do it deliberately. Some parents make the mistake of thinking their children can control their bladders when they choose to because they have managed to stay dry while staying with a friend or relative. In fact, this is usually because children tend to sleep more lightly in unfamiliar surroundings and so they wake more easily. In some cases, children deliberately stay awake for most of the night to avoid the embarrassment of wetting while at a friend's house.

Education and Resources for Improving Childhood Continence (ERIC) is a very useful organization which provides information, advice and practical support for parents and children who are affected.

Visit their website at <www.eric.org.uk> or see p. 109 for contact details.

Growing pains

Many people still think that the idea of 'growing pains' is an old wives' tale. This is probably because there is no scientific reason or any firm evidence why the growth of bones, joints or muscles should cause pain. However, if you have an otherwise healthy child who wakes night after night screaming that his or her legs hurt, you'll be in no doubt that the condition does exist! Growing pains are most common between the ages of four and 12. We don't know why some children experience these pains, which are usually in the legs, but it has been suggested that they may be due to strain on the muscles attached to growing bones. These muscles may tire easily, causing pain at night when they finally relax.

If your child wakes in the night with pains in the legs, check first that there is no obvious cause, such as a previously unnoticed injury. Is there any swelling or redness in the area or around the joints? Does movement increase the pain? Can your child point to the exact area and if so, is it tender to the touch? Does your child have a fever or any unexplained rash? If any of these apply, you should consult a doctor to establish the cause. If not, it's likely your child has growing pains. It may be difficult for your child to identify exactly where the pain is, but it can be in one leg or both, and can last from a few minutes up to an hour or more. It can sometimes be quite severe, but is always gone by the morning. Sometimes, the pain causes the child to tighten his or her leg muscles, which can trigger cramp, in turn causing residual soreness in the morning.

The most effective way to deal with growing pains seems to be to rub the affected areas to relieve the discomfort. Often the pain goes after a few minutes and the child goes back to sleep easily. If the pain is prolonged, it may be worth giving a junior analgesic of some kind. Most children grow out of growing pains by the time they reach their teens.

Anxiety

Just like adults, children can also be kept awake by stress, worry and anxiety. If your child has difficulty going to sleep or wakes in the night and cannot get back to sleep and you can't find any obvious reason, it may be that he or she is anxious about something. If there is something going on at home or school that you're aware of, it may help your child to talk about this so that you can offer comfort and reassurance. If there's nothing obvious, try asking gently about things that may be a source of worry. Are there problems at school? Has she fallen out with a friend? Is he concerned about a relative? Is there something he's frightened of? There may be a very simple and easily dealt with reason.

If your child has ongoing sleep difficulties that you cannot resolve, his or her schooling and general health is likely to be affected, so do talk to your doctor or health visitor about the situation.

Final word

Whether your nights are disturbed by wakeful children, snoring partners or noisy neighbours, or whether you simply lie awake for hours for no apparent reason, I hope you have found some useful information and advice in this book. Insomnia can make you feel irritable, bleak and lonely – as well as tired. But it can also give you an opportunity to see things other people only hear about: the Milky Way in a clear night sky; a twinkling of frost in the moonlight; the magic of dawn breaking on the horizon. On those few occasions when you've tried everything and you still can't sleep, try not to worry; enjoy the peace, beauty and tranquillity of the early hours, and remember, you will sleep eventually.

Useful addresses

Age Concern
Astral House
1268 London Road
London SW16 4ER
Helpline: 0800 00 99 66 (8 a.m. to 7 p.m., seven days a week)
Website: www.ageconcern.org.uk

Many useful fact sheets available; separate offices in Northern Ireland, Scotland and Wales.

Allergy UK
3 White Oak Square
London Road
Swanley
Kent BR8 7AG
Helpline: 01322 619 898
Website: www.allergyuk.org

Association of Reflexologists
5 Fore Street
Taunton
Somerset TA1 1HX
Tel.: 0870 567 3320
Website: www.aor.org.uk

British Acupuncture Council
63 Jeddo Road
London W12 9HQ
Tel.: 020 8735 0400
Website: www.acupuncture.org.uk

British Association for Counselling and Psychotherapy (BACP)
BACP House
15 St John's Business Park
Lutterworth
Leicestershire LE17 4HB
Tel.: 0870 443 5252
Website: www.bacp.co.uk

British Snoring and Sleep Apnoea Association (BSSAA)
Castle Court
41 London Road
Reigate RH2 9RJ
Tel.: 01737 245638
Website: www.britishsnoring.co.uk

British Wheel of Yoga
BWY Central Office
25 Jermyn Street
Sleaford
Lincolnshire NG34 7RU
Tel.: 01529 306851
Website: www.bwy.org.uk

Centre for Anxiety Disorders and Trauma
99 Denmark Hill
London SE5 8AF
Tel.: 020 3228 2101/3286
Website: http://psychology.iop.kcl.ac.uk

Citizens Advice Bureau
Website: www.citizensadvice.org,uk

Clinical Sleep Research Unit
Department of Human Sciences
Loughborough University
Leicestershire LE11 3TU
Tel.: 01509 222288
Website: www.lboro.ac.uk

Cruse Bereavement Care
PO Box 800
Richmond
Surrey TW9 1RG
Helpline: 0844 477 9400
Website: www.crusebereavementcare.org.uk

Cry-sis Helpline
BM Cry-sis
London WC1 3XX
Tel.: 08451 228 669
Website: www.cry-sis.org.uk

Provides support for parents whose babies cry excessively.

Education and Resources for Improving Childhood Continence (ERIC)
34 Old School House
Britannia Road
Kingswood
Bristol BS15 8DB
Tel.: 0845 370 8008 (10 a.m. to 4 p.m., Monday to Friday)
Website: www.eric.org.uk

Ekbom Support Group
C/o 42 Nursery Road
Rainham
Gillingham
Kent ME8 0BE

A support group for those with restless legs syndrome.

The International Federation of Professional Aromatherapists (IFPA)
82 Ashby Road
Hinckley
Leicestershire LE10 1SN
Tel.: 01455 637987
Website: www.ifparoma.org

International Stress Management Association
PO Box 26
South Petherton TA13 5WY
Tel.: 07000 780430
Website: www.isma.org.uk

Lumie
3 The Links
Trafalgar Way
Bar Hill
Cambridge CB23 8UD
Tel.: 01954 780 500
Website: www.lumie.com

A firm providing supplies in the field of light therapy for those with seasonal affective disorder (SAD) or similar.

Narcolepsy Association UK (UKAN)
PO Box 13842
Penicuik EH26 8WX
Tel.: 0845 450 0394
Website: www.narcolepsy.org.uk

National Debtline
Tel.: 0808 808 4000
Website: www.nationaldebtline.co.uk

National Institute of Medical Herbalists
Elm House
54 Mary Arches Street
Exeter EX4 3BA
Tel.: 01392 426022
Website: www.nimh.org.uk

Relate
Carolina Court
Lakeside
Doncaster DN4 5RA
Tel.: 0845 456 1310
Relate response line: 0845 130 4016 (8 a.m. to 10 p.m., Monday to
Thursday, 8 a.m. to 5 p.m., Friday and Saturday, midday to 5 p.m.,
Sunday)
Website: www.relate.org.uk

The Royal Society for the Prevention of Accidents (RoSPA)
RoSPA House
Edgbaston Park
353 Bristol Road
Edgbaston
Birmingham B5 7ST
Tel.: 0121 248 2000
Website: www.rospa.com

Sleep Apnoea Scotland
26 Sinclair Way
Livingston
West Lothian EH54 8HW
Website: www.scottishsleepapnoea.co.uk

The Sleep Apnoea Trust (SATA)
2a Bakers Piece
Kingston Blount
Oxon OX39 4SW
Tel.: 0845 60 60 685
Website: www.sleep-apnoea-trust.org

The Sleep Council
High Corn Mill
Chapel Hill
Skipton
North Yorkshire BD23 1NL
Freephone leaflet line: 0800 018 2923
Insomnia helpline: 020 8994 9874 (6 p.m. to 8 p.m., Monday to Friday)
Website: www.sleepcouncil.com

The Sleep Paralysis Information Service
C/o Fourmiles Media Services
PO Box 5571
Milton Keynes MK3 5YN
Tel.: 0709 222 3643
Website: www.spis.org.uk

Society of Homeopaths
11 Brookfield
Duncan Close
Moulton Park
Northampton NN3 6WL
Tel.: 0845 450 6611
Website: www.homeopathy-soh.org

Welsh Sleep Apnoea Society
2 Greenfield Close
Pontnewydd
Cwmbran NP44 1BY
Helpline: 01633 774087
Website: www.welshsas.org

The helpline is not allowed to give medical advice.

Further reading

Branch, Rhena, and Wilson, Rob, *Cognitive Behaviour Therapy Workbook for Dummies*. John Wiley & Sons, Chichester, 2007.

Courtin, Robina, and McDonald, Kathleen, *How to Meditate*. Wisdom Publications, Somerville, Massachusetts, 2005.

Davies, Dr Dilys, *Insomnia: Your Questions Answered*. Vega, London, 2002.

Deits, Bob, *Life after Loss – A Practical Guide to Renewing Your Life after a Major Loss*. Da Capo Press, Cambridge, Massachusetts, 2004.

Espie, Colin A., *Overcoming Insomnia and Sleep Problems: A Self-Help Guide Using Cognitive Behavioral Techniques*. Constable & Robinson, London, 2006.

Gilbert, Paul, *Overcoming Depression*. Constable & Robinson, London, 2000.

Harrison, Yvonne, *Sleep Talking: Science Needs and Misconceptions*. Blandford, Poole, 1999.

Idizikowski, Chris, *Beating Insomnia: How to Get a Good Night's Sleep*. Newleaf, Bremen, 2003.

Illman, John, *Use Your Brain to Beat Depression*. Cassell Illustrated, London, 2004.

Lader, Malcolm, *Tranquillizers and Antidepressants: When to Start Them, How to Stop*. Sheldon Press, London, 2008.

Riha, Dr Renata L. *Sleep – Your Questions Answered*. Dorling Kindersley, London, 2007.

Van Straten, Michael, *The Good Sleep Guide*. Kyle Cathie Limited, London, 2004.

Index